FIGHT KIDNEY DISEASE & DIABETES

SIMPLE AND PRACTICAL REAL LIFE STRATEGIES TO HELP IMPROVE CHRONIC KIDNEY DISEASE & DIABETIC PATIENTS' QUALITY OF LIFE THROUGH DIET!

KidneyBuzz.com

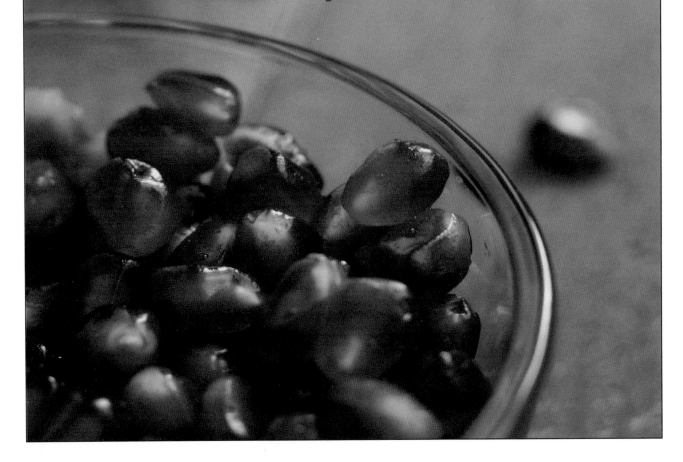

Notes

To KidneyBuzz.com Viewers: Everything we do, we do with you in mind. Here's to LIFE!

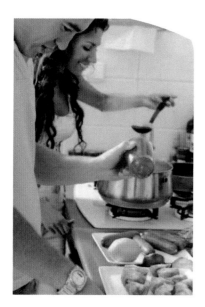

Introduction

Fight Kidney Disease and Diabetes, details easy to implement healthy and tasty Renal and Diabetic-Friendly recipes. This book provides practical advice on physical, mental and emotional stability - all of which can assist you in living longer and better.

The KidneyBuzz.com Team would like to extend a BIG Thank You to our many viewers who requested that we write a more extensive guide after our free "KidneyBuzz.com Impact Meals" Volume I. We have created, "Fight Kidney Disease and Diabetes," to help you take your diet, whether Renal or Diabetic, to the next level because you are at the heart and soul of everything we do.

KidneyBuzz.com Impact Meals, was the first recipe book of its kind tailored to the holistic needs of the Chronic Kidney Disease (CKD) Community and offered free of charge. Many readers told us that they appreciated the comprehensiveness of that book. They encouraged us to make this second edition that will be even more useful for our readers including those with Diabetes who represent more than 43% of the CKD patients. This guide retained the highly practical, easily understandable and concise content of the first. But, it also contains significant changes that came about as a result of constructive suggestions from many of our supporters who are also healthcare professionals.

For more information about our other products or Renal and Diabetic tailored Daily News coverage, you can visit KidneyBuzz.com

KIDNEYBUZZ.COM TEAM

Published By: The United Network (America)

21520 Yorba Linda Blvd. G238
Yorba Linda, CA 92887

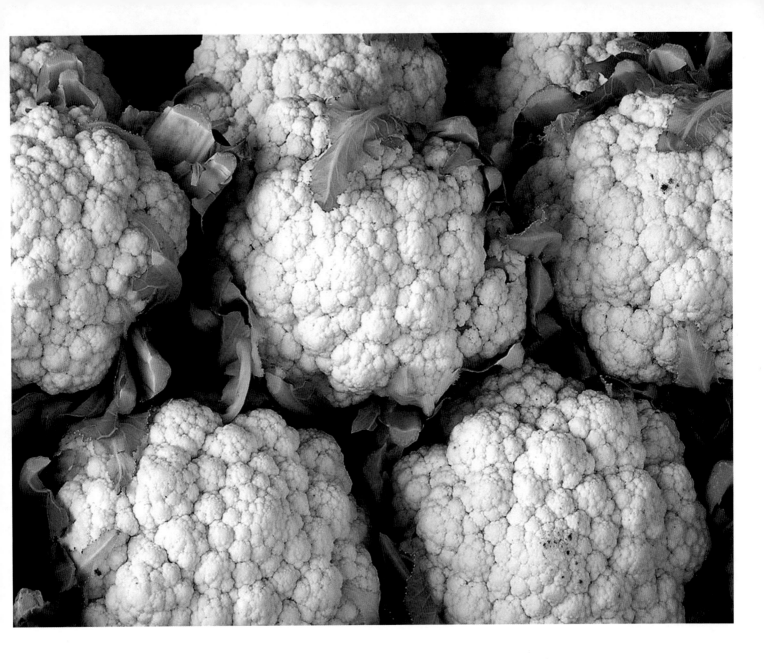

Cauliflower

The health benefits of cauliflower are huge for Chronic Kidney Disease patients and Diabetics. It is not a vegetable in the traditional sense. When you eat Cauliflower, you are actually eating the flower of the plant which provides several important nutrients including vitamin C, vitamin K, your daily recommended intake of vitamin B6, calcium and iron. This treat is low in phosphorus and potassium which is good for CKD patients in balancing their mineral levels. Cauliflower also encourages bodily cells to increase enzymes which detoxifies the body of harmful chemicals. Studies have linked this flower to protection from cancer and rheumatoid arthritis. At only $1.42 per pound you can afford to incorporate Cauliflower into your regular diet.

Balsamic & Parmesan Roasted Cauliflower

INGREDIENTS	QUANTITY
Cauliflower Florets	8 Cups
Extra-Virgin Olive Oil	2 Tablespoons
Dried Marjoram	1 Teaspoon
Salt	1/4 Teaspoon
Balsamic Vinegar	2 Tablespoons
Finely Shredded Parmesan Cheese	1/2 Cup
Freshly Ground Pepper	To Taste

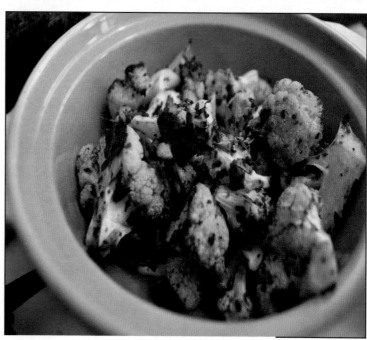

Image courtesy of ohbernadine/http://www.photoree.com/

PREPARATION

1. Preheat oven to 450°F.
2. Toss cauliflower, oil, marjoram, salt and pepper in a large bowl.
3. Spread on a large rimmed baking sheet and roast until starting to soften and brown on the bottom, 15 to 20 minutes.
4. Toss the cauliflower with vinegar and sprinkle with cheese.
5. Return to the oven and roast until the cheese is melted and any moisture has evaporated, 5 to 10 minutes more.

Tip: To prepare florets from a whole head of cauliflower, remove outer leaves. Slice off the thick stem. With the head upside down and holding a knife at a 45° angle, slice into the smaller stems with a circular motion—removing a "plug" from the center of the head. Break or cut florets into the desired size.

NUTRITION INFORMATION PER SERVING

Serving 4
Calories - 149
Protein - 7g.
Carbohydrate - 10g.
Total Fat - 10g.
Trans Fat - 0g.
Cholesterol - 7mg.
Potassium - 180mg.
Sodium - 260mg.
Phosphorus - 40mg.
Sugars - 0g.

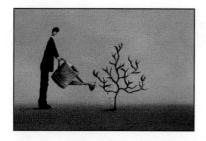

PITFALLS OF RENAL DIET

The renal diet may take some time for you to learn to follow. If you do not eat enough food, you may not get the calories, protein, and other nutrients that your body needs. You may lose weight. If you do not follow a renal diet, your kidneys will work harder. This may cause total renal failure to happen sooner. If you have total renal failure, then properly following this diet will be critical to improving your quality of life.

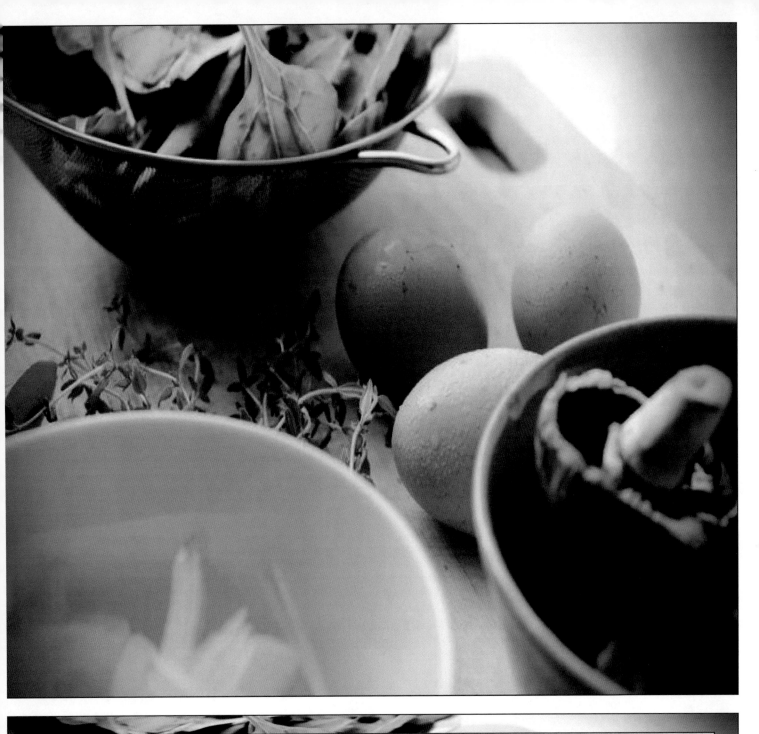

Chicken & Mushroom

Although many Physicians and Dietitians often recommend a diet that is low protein and fat, Medical Xpress reported on January 15th, 2014 that obese people with diabetes are able to lose weight through high-protein diets and, in fact, see improvements in both cardiovascular and renal health, despite initial concerns about the impact on their renal health.

Chicken Breasts with Mushroom Cream Sauce

INGREDIENTS	QUANTITY
Chicken Breasts (Boneless; Skinless)	2 Breasts
Freshly Ground Pepper	1/2 Tablespoon
Salt	1/4 Teaspoon
Canola Oil	1 Teaspoon
Shallot	1 Medium
Shiitake Mushroom Caps (Thinly Sliced)	1 Cup
Dry Vermouth or Dry White Wine (Optional)	2 Tablespoons
Reduced-sodium Chicken Broth	1/4 Cup
Heavy Cream	2 Tablespoons
Minced Fresh Chives or Scallion Greens	2 Tablespoons

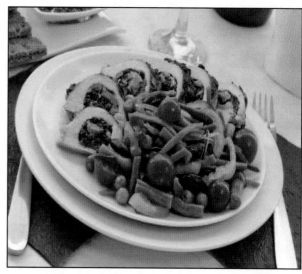

Image courtesy of Apolonia / http://www.freedigitalphotos.net/

PREPARATION

1. Season chicken with pepper and salt on both sides.
2. Heat oil in a medium skillet over medium heat.
3. Add the chicken and cook, turning once or twice and adjusting the heat to prevent burning, until brown and an instant-read thermometer inserted into the thickest part registers 165°F, 12 to 16 minutes.
4. Transfer to a plate and tent with foil to keep warm.
5. Add shallot to the pan and cook, stirring, until fragrant, about 30 seconds.
6. Add mushrooms; cook, stirring occasionally until tender, about 2 minutes.
7. Pour in vermouth (or wine); simmer until almost evaporated, scraping up any browned bits, about 1 minute.
8. Pour in broth and cook until reduced by half, 1 to 2 minutes.
9. Stir in cream and chives (or scallions); return to a simmer.
10. Return the chicken to the pan, turn to coat with sauce and cook until heated through, about 1 minute.

Tip: It's difficult to find an individual chicken breast small enough for one portion. Removing the thin strip of meat from the underside of a 5-ounce breast—the "tender"—removes about 1 ounce of meat and yields a perfect 4-ounce portion. Wrap and freeze the tenders and when you have gathered enough, use them in a stir-fry or for oven-baked chicken fingers.

NUTRITION INFORMATION PER SERVING

Serves 2
Calories - 274
Protein - 25g.
Carbohydrate - 5g.
Total Fat - 15g.
Trans Fat - 0g.
Cholesterol - 83mg.
Potassium - 105mg.
Sodium - 125mg.
Phosphorus - 60mg.
Sugars - 0g.

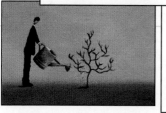

KIDNEY FAILURE AND DIABETES

According to the United States Renal Data System, the primary cause of Kidney Failure was Diabetes for 43.8% of Chronic Kidney Disease (CKD) patients. What is worse, Medpage.com notes that nearly 90% of type II Diabetes patients may be living with CKD and go completely undiagnosed (22% in CKD stages 3-5).

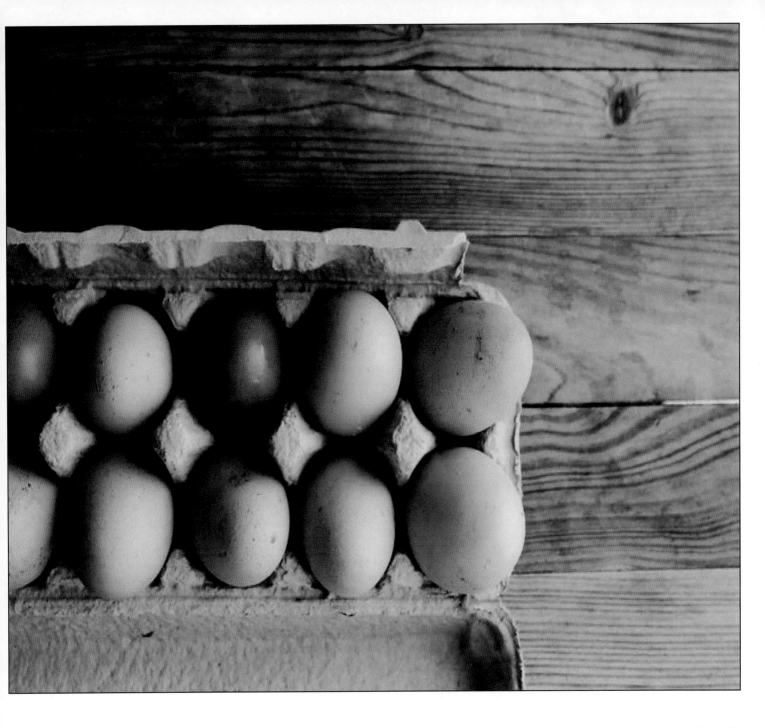

Are You Chicken?

Often overlooked, Dialysis and Diabetic patients usually need to incorporate high-quality proteins into their diet to avoid becoming sluggish, tired and decrease their risk for infections. While your Dietitian may recommend energy or protein supplements when your protein levels are low, they can become quite expensive, and add to your medication burden. What's more is by eating lean meat such as chicken you can improve your protein levels as well as your overall health.

Sautéed Chicken and Steamed Asparagus

INGREDIENT	QUANTITY
Trimmed And Cut Asparagus	8 Ounces
Reduced-Sodium Chicken Broth	2/3 Cup
All-Purpose Flour	1/4 Cup
Boneless and Skinless Chicken Breasts	1 1/4 to 1 1/2 Pounds
Freshly Ground Pepper	1/2 Teaspoon
Canola Oil (Olive Oil Optional)	1 Tablespoon
Thinly Sliced Shallot	1 Shallot
White Wine (optional)	1/2 Cup
Reduced-Fat Sour Cream	1/3 Cup
Chopped Fresh Tarragon	1 Tablespoon
Lemon Juice	2 Teaspoons
Shredded Gruyère Cheese	2/3 Cup

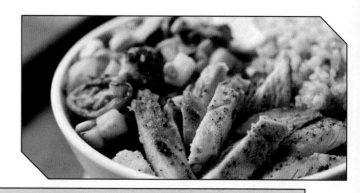

NUTRITION INFORMATION PER SERVING
Serves 4
Calories - 204
Protein - 31g.
Carbohydrate - 7g.
Total Fat - 14g.
Trans Fat - 0g.
Cholesterol - 90mg.
Potassium - 250mg.
Sodium - 267mg.
Phosphorus - 95mg.
Sugars - 0g.

PREPARATION
1. Place a steamer basket in a large saucepan, add 1 inch of water and bring to a boil.
2. Add asparagus; cover and steam for 3 minutes.
3. Uncover, remove from the heat and set aside.
4. Whisk broth and 2 teaspoons flour in a small bowl until smooth. Set aside.
5. Place the remaining 1/4 cup flour in a shallow dish.
6. Sprinkle chicken with pepper and dredge both sides in the flour, shaking off any excess.
7. Heat oil in a large skillet over medium heat.
8. Add the chicken and cook until golden brown, 3 to 4 minutes per side, adjusting heat as needed to prevent scorching.
9. Transfer to a plate and cover to keep warm.
10. Add shallot, wine and the reserved broth mixture to the pan; cook over medium heat, stirring, until thickened, about 2 minutes.
11. Reduce heat to medium-low; stir in sour cream, tarragon, lemon juice and the reserved asparagus until combined.
12. Return the chicken to the pan and turn to coat with the sauce.
13. Sprinkle cheese on top of each piece of chicken, cover and continue cooking until the cheese is melted, about 2 minutes.
Note: You can substitute the white wine in recipe for a non-alcoholic wine or remove it entirely. Also, forgo cheese if it conflicts with your renal or diabetic diet.

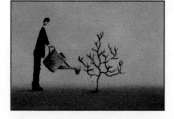

FLUID INTAKE
Most hemodialysis patients are restricted to no more than 40oz of fluid within 24 hrs which means they should only gain 2-3kg between treatments. If you stick to this rule, it may go a long way toward making you feel better during and after treatments.
More Fluid > Larger Fluid Withdraw Goals > Harder Treatment On Your Body

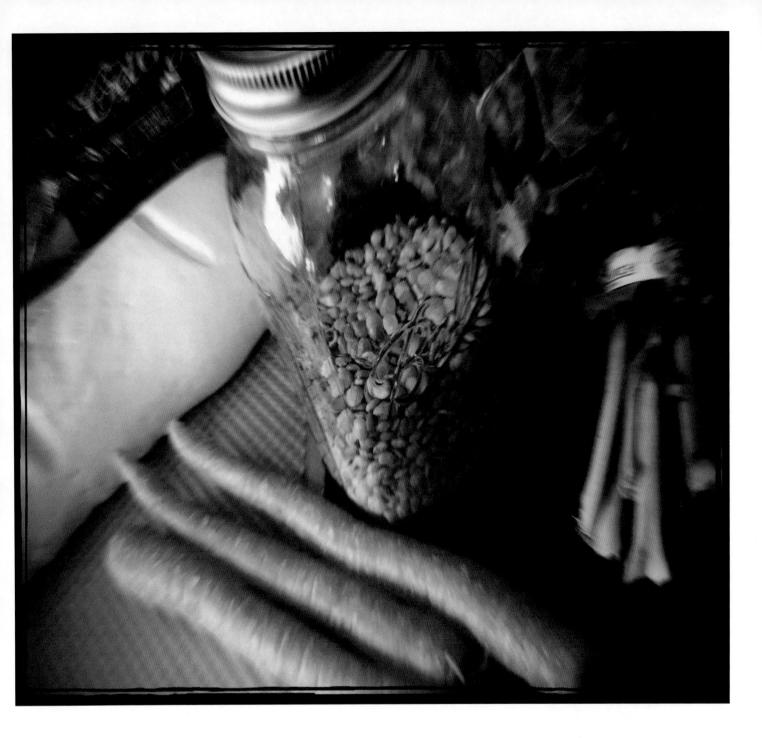

Fresh Vegetable Purée

New research presented to the American Society of Nephrology in November 2013 shows that increasing consumption of vegetable protein is linked with prolonged survival among people who have Chronic Kidney Disease (CKD) and Diabetes because vegetable protein intake produces less harmful toxins when compared with meat protein.

Seasoned Creamy Cauliflower Purée

INGREDIENTS	QUANTITY
Bite-Size Cauliflower Florets	8 Cup (About One Head)
Crushed and Peeled Garlic	4 Cloves
Buttermilk	1/3 Cup
Extra-Virgin Olive Oil	4 Tablespoons
Butter	1 Teaspoon
Salt (Optional)	1/2 Teaspoon
Freshly Ground Pepper	To Taste
Snipped Fresh Chives for Garnish	

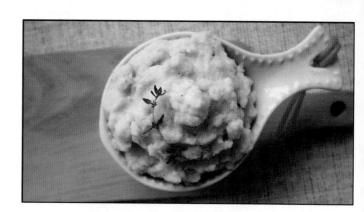

NUTRITION INFORMATION PER SERVING
Serves 4
Calories - 108
Protein - 4g.
Carbohydrate - 10g.
Total Fat - 7g.
Trans Fat - 0g.
Cholesterol - 3mg.
Potassium - 180mg.
Sodium - 342mg.
Phosphorus - 40mg.
Sugars - 0g.

PREPARATION

1. Place cauliflower florets and garlic in a steamer basket over boiling water, cover and steam until very tender, 12 to 15 minutes. (Alternatively, place florets and garlic in a microwave-safe bowl with 1/4 cup water, cover and microwave on High for 3 to 5 minutes.)
2. Place the cooked cauliflower and garlic in a food processor.
3. Add buttermilk, 2 teaspoons oil, butter, salt and pepper; pulse several times, then process until smooth and creamy.
4. Transfer to a serving bowl. Drizzle with the remaining 2 teaspoons oil and garnish with chives, if desired. Serve hot.

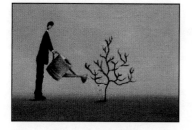

REDUCING HEART ATTACK RISK

Although Doctors usually tell their Chronic Kidney Disease (CKD) and Diabetic patients that walking is beneficial for them, new research published in the journal, Lancet, provides a concrete number. By walking 2000 steps each day which is the equivalent of 20 minutes of moderate paced walking or walking one mile, an individual can lower their risk of a heart attack by 8%.

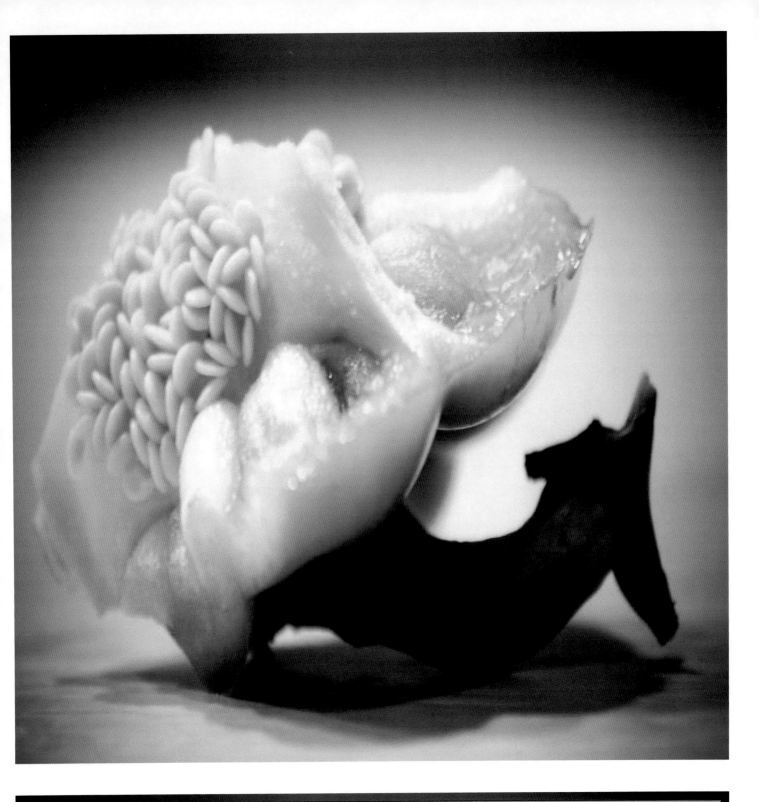

Eating Your Greens

Gardening can be tailored therapy to the specific needs and abilities of the individual gardener; improving the body, lifting the spirits, as well as stimulating the mind. Working with plants have been proven to increase movement and minimize depression for people with Diabetes and Chronic Kidney Disease. Hence, producing your own vegetables would not only help to reduce your food budget, but will also encourage you to eat healthy, and be active.

Cabbage and Beef Stew

INGREDIENTS	QUANTITY
Beef Blade Steaks	2 Pounds
Cold Water	6 Cups
Olive Oil	2 Tablespoons
Low-Sodium Tomato Sauce	1/2 Cups
Cabbage	1 Medium Head
Onion	1 Cup
Carrots	1 Cup
Turnips	1 Cup
Lemon Juice	6 Tablespoons

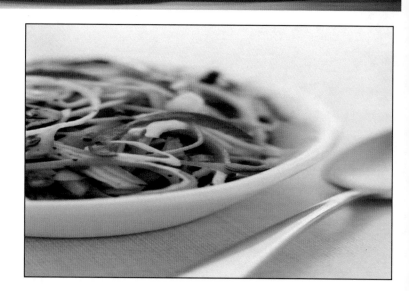

PREPARATION

1. Place steak in a big pot.
2. Add water to cover meat completely.
3. Cover with lid and bring to a boil.
4. After water is boiling, reduce heat to simmer and cook until meat is tender and shreds easily.
5. Remove meat from pot and shred with a fork.
6. Cut cabbage into bite-size pieces. Peel and dice onion, carrots and turnips.
7. Leave water in pot and add olive oil, tomato sauce, cabbage, onion, carrots, turnips and shredded meat.
8. Season with salt and pepper; add lemon juice and sugar.
9. Cook on low heat 1 to 1-1/2 hours until all vegetables are cooked.
10. Before serving season to taste with more lemon, sugar or pepper if desired.
Note: You can opt not to use beef and substitute it for chicken or go meatless entirely. It is still a great dish!

NUTRITION INFORMATION PER SERVING

Serves 12
Calories - 202
Protein - 19g.
Carbohydrate - 9g.
Total Fat - 10g.
Trans Fat - 0g.
Cholesterol - 60mg.
Potassium - 0mg.
Sodium - 242mg.
Phosphorus - 50mg.
Sugars - 0g.

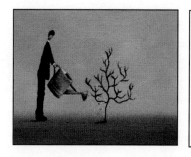

VEGATABLES THAT HYDRATE

A new study has found that some watery fruits and vegetables such as cabbage may hydrate the body twice as effectively as a glass of water, making them a refreshing snack option that can help to decrease fluid intake, as well as help those with CKD and Diabetes feel fuller longer, make them less likely to snack on unhealthy foods, and serve as a main component of a low-fat and low-calorie diet. Other nutrient-rich vegetables with high water content include broccoli, cauliflower, eggplant and spinach.

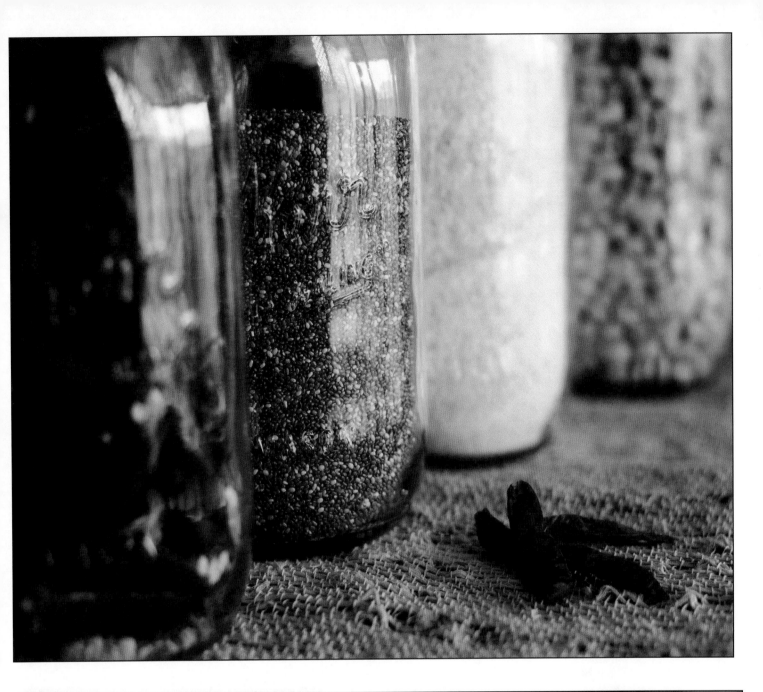

Spice It Up!

To stay healthy, control their blood pressure and protect their kidney health, people with Diabetes and Chronic Kidney Disease have to control their levels of salt, potassium, phosphorus, and saturated fats by limiting their intake of certain foods. You do not have to settle for food that is boring or bland. By using chili powder, lemon zest, dried oregano, smoked paprika and Italian Seasoning, you can spice up any meal!

Image courtesy of Nomadic Lass/http://www.flickr.com/

Easy and Delicious Kebabs

INGREDIENTS	QUANTITY
Top Sirloin Steak (also substitute fish, chicken and vegetarian)	1 1/2 Pounds
Bell Pepper	1 Large
Red Onions	2 Medium
Button Mushrooms	1/2 Pounds
Bamboo or Wooden Skewers	20 Skewers
Olive Oil	1/3 Cup
Soy Sauce	1/3 Cup
Red Wine Vinegar	3 Tablespoons
Honey	1/4 Cup
Minced Garlic	2 Cloves
Minced Fresh Ginger	1 Tablespoon
Freshly Ground Black	To Taste

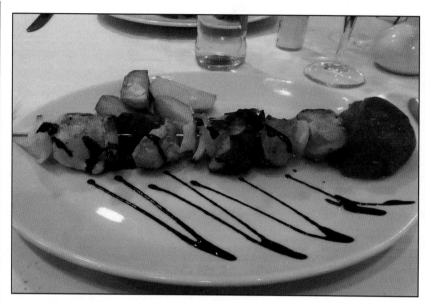

Image courtesy of Karen V Bryan / http://www.flickr.com/

PREPARATION

1. Mix the marinade ingredients together in a bowl and add the meat.
2. Cover and chill in the fridge for at least 30 minutes, preferably several hours or even overnight.
3. Soak the skewers in water for at least 30 minutes before grilling.
4. This will help prevent them from completely burning up on the grill.
5. Cut the vegetables into chunks roughly the width of the beef pieces.
6. Taking care not to poke yourself, thread the meat and vegetables onto double bamboo skewers.
7. One way to do this safely is to put the piece that you are trying to pierce on a cutting board, and then push the skewers through the piece to the board.
8. Using double skewers will help you turn the kebabs on the grill.
9. If you keep a little space between the pieces, they will grill more evenly.
10. Paint the kebabs with some of the remaining marinade.
11. Prepare your grill for high, direct heat.
12. Grill for 8 to 10 minutes, depending on how hot your grill is, and how done you would like your meat, turning occasionally.
Let rest for 5 minutes before serving.

NUTRITION INFORMATION PER SERVING

Serves 6
Calories - 194
Protein - 6g.
Carbohydrate - 10g.
Total Fat - 6g.
Trans Fat - 0g.
Cholesterol - 14mg.
Potassium - 50mg.
Sodium - 170mg.
Phosphorus - 70mg.
Sugars - 0g.

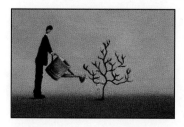

EATING WELL ON A BUDGET

These tough economic times should remind those living on a fixed budget about the importance of pinching pennies. But what does that really mean for people suffering with Chronic Kidney Disease (CKD)and diabetes who have to be concerned with eating healthy as well? KidneyBuzz.com suggests you can accomplish both. You can Eat For Less while Eating Healthy! Learn how.

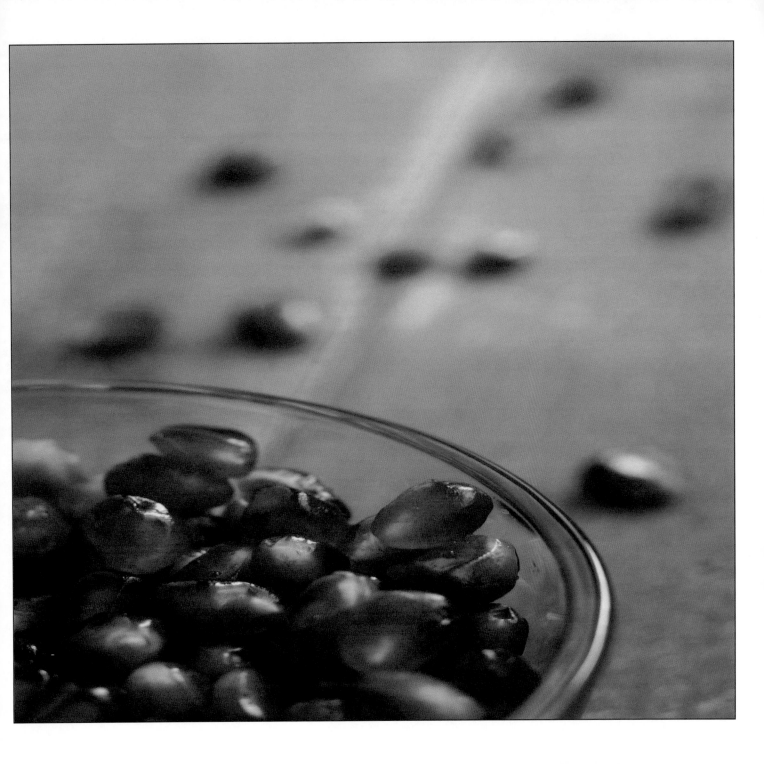

Avoiding Temptation

Choosing foods that are from the main food groups such as whole grains, low fat dairy vegetables, fruit, and protein will help you stay healthy and avoid consuming meals that contain excess sugar and salt.

Image courtesy of Nomadic Lass/http://www.flickr.com/

Fun Quiz: What Your Cravings Reveal About You

At one time or another most Chronic Kidney Disease (CKD) and Diabetic patients have sugar and salt cravings and generally there is no apparent cause for concern if you do not indulge the cravings. However, I never considered that our different eating habits could coincide with our different personalities. But according to Alan R. Hirsch, M.D., head of the Smell & Taste Research Center in Chicago, eating habits are related to character traits. The old saying is reinforced, "You are what you eat!" A study suggests that there are some consistent generalizations of what food choices and cravings say about our personality. Take the quiz below and find out whether you are sweet or salty and what that means for your treatment plan.

1.) What is a better dinner for you?
a. Barbecue Chicken
b. Steak

2.) What would you prefer to snack on at the movies?
a. Popcorn
b. Candy

3.) What would you prefer to have with a bagged lunch?
a. Potato Chips
b. A Cookie

4.) What would you prefer to have for breakfast?
a. Pancakes
b. Eggs and Bacon

5.) What side salad would you prefer?
a. Fruit Salad
b. Garden Salad

6.) What sandwich would you prefer for lunch?
a. Grilled Cheese
b. Peanut Butter and Jelly

7.) What would you rather put on your toast?
a. Butter
b. Jam

8.) Which piece of pie would you rather end the night with?
a. A Slice of Apple Pie
b. A Slice of Pizza Pie

9.) How do you take your coffee or tea?
a. Black
b. With Sugar/Cream

Salty: If you chose mostly A's then you enjoy salty foods. Besides salty snacks, it is also likely that you go for something with a bit of crunch, zest, or spice. Unlike those that like sweets, you "go with the flow," take things in stride, and likely believe that "what will be, will be" and thus your fate is out of your hands. You may tend to crave salt when times are stressful or tense. Consider a healthier fix to maintain your Renal/Diabetic diet such as veggies with hummus. Also, experimenting with different herbs and spices can add savor to your food that is often missing when sodium is restricted. Be careful with cuisines that rely on soy sauce, miso and black bean paste to flavor foods because these are invariably high in sodium.

Sweet: If you chose mostly B's then sweets are your preferred choice. When it comes to snack time you are much more likely to grab something sweet rather than salty. Your personality is generally agreeable and kind. You are actually sweet. Sweet foods are known to bring comfort so you may seek them out when you feel the need for a bit of pampering. When sugary treats are consumed often it encourages weight gain and can cause harmful health side-effects. For a healthier sugar fix, substitute candy and chocolate with fresh fruit. Fruit has natural sugars that will help satisfy a sweet craving while helping you maintain healthy eating habits.

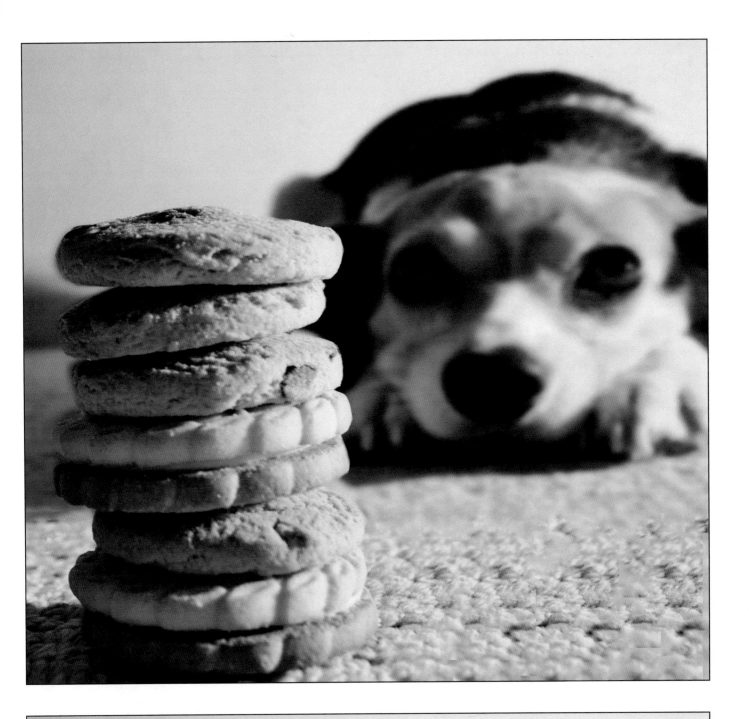

Enjoying The Journey

For those with a sweet tooth, fresh fruit that is low in potassium (apples, strawberries, pineapple, grapes and plums) can make for an excellent treat and you can even enjoy it with sugar-free whipped topping while maintaining a healthy renal/diabetic diet. Also, Livestrong.com suggests that sugar-free gelatin and ice pops are other good sweet snack ideas as long as you count them toward your daily fluid intake. Animal crackers, vanilla wafers and graham crackers are kidney-friendly snacks that you can include in moderation but may contribute high amounts of carbohydrates if you do not control portions.

No Sugar Sugar-Cookies

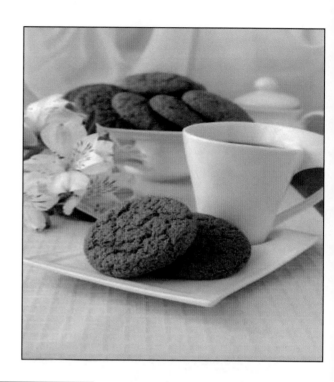

INGREDIENTS	QUANTITY
Unsalted Butter	3/4 Cups
Light Butter	1/4 Cups
Splenda or Stevia	1 Cup
Vanilla	1 Tablespoon
Eggs	1/4 Cup
Water	1/4 Cup
Vinegar	3/4 Teaspoon
All Purpose Flour (Almond Flour as Substitute)	1 1/2 Cups
Cake Flour	1 1/2 Cups
Salt	1/4 Teaspoons
Baking Powder	1 Teaspoon

PREPARATION
1. Preheat oven to 350 degrees F. Lightly oil a cookie sheet and set aside.
2. Blend together butters, Splenda Granulated Sweetener and vanilla in a medium mixing bowl with an electric mixer, or by hand.
3. Blend until butter is softened. Add egg substitute, water and vinegar.
4. Mix briefly. Add flours, salt and baking powder. Mix on low speed, until dough is formed. Do not over-mix.
5. Remove dough from bowl and place on a floured work surface. Divide dough in half. Pat each half into a circle and cover with plastic wrap.
6. Refrigerate approx. 1 hour, allowing dough to chill.
7. Remove dough from refrigerator and roll out on a floured work surface to desired thickness, approx. 1/4 inch. Cut with cookie cutters. Place cookies on prepared sheet.
8. Bake in a preheated 350 degrees F oven 10-12 minutes or until lightly browned on the back. Cool on a wire rack.

NUTRITION INFORMATION PER SERVING
Serves 48
Calories - 60
Protein - 1g.
Carbohydrate - 7g.
Total Fat - 3g.
Trans Fat - 0g.
Cholesterol - 10mg.
Potassium - 40mg.
Sodium - 30mg.
Phosphorus - 58mg.
Sugars - 1g.

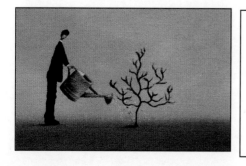

SNACKING RIGHT
Snacks that you can eat include unsalted breadsticks or pretzels, air-popped popcorn seasoned with a sodium-free herb blend, and Melba toast with light cream cheese. You may also enjoy cut-up fresh vegetables, such as celery sticks, cucumbers, carrots and cauliflower with a low-fat salad dressing for dipping. As you likely know, if you have CKD and/or Diabetes, you should still avoid food with any visible salt sprinkles, chocolate, or nuts.

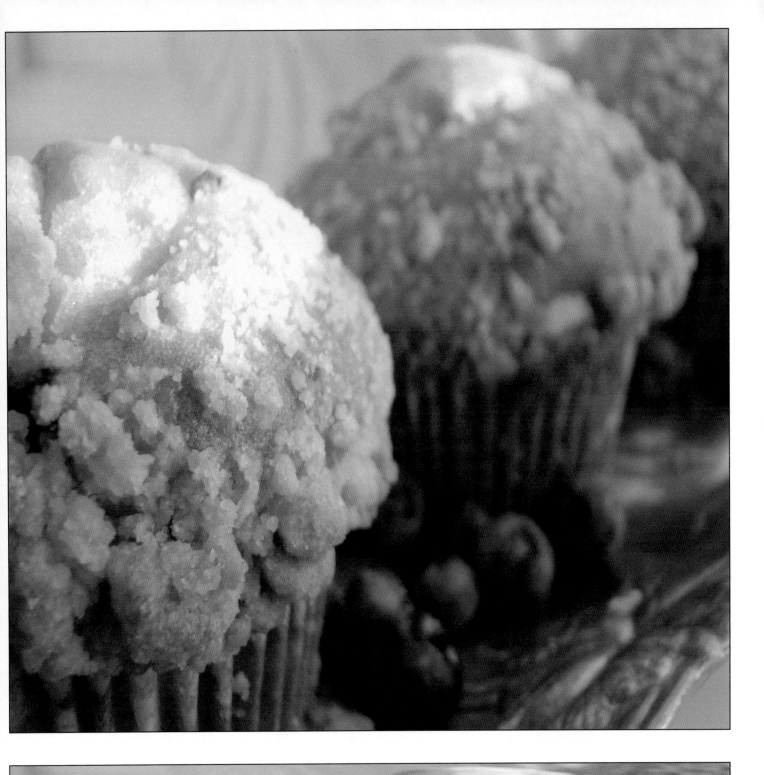

Benefits Of Berries

According to research from Harvard University, eating three servings of blueberries a week can cut the risk of having a heart attack by one third. This is because blueberries contain the super antioxidant dietary compounds called Anthocyanins.

Low-Carb Loaded Blueberry and Oat Muffins

INGREDIENTS	QUANTITY
Almond Flour	1 Cup
Dry Quick Cooking Oats	1/2 Cup
Sugar (Stevia Optional)	1/2 Cup
Baking Powder	1 Teaspoon
Baking Soda	1/2 Teaspoon
Salt	1/4 Teaspoon
Egg Whites	2 Large
Water	1/2 Cup
Olive Oil	1/3 Cup
Frozen or Fresh Blueberries	1 Cup
Sugar	2 Tablespoons
Cinnamon	1/4 Teaspoons

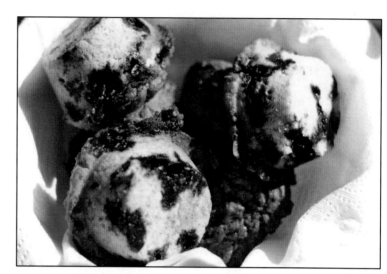

Image courtesy of rudy.kleysteuber/photoree.com

PREPARATION DIRECTIONS
1. Preheat the oven to 400 degrees Fahrenheit.
2. Line 12 muffin cups with paper baking cups.
3. Mix 6 six ingredients in a bowl to distribute baking soda and salt.
4. In a second bowl beat the egg whites, water and oil.
5. Stir into the dry ingredients until just moistened, batter will be lumpy.
6. Fold in blueberries.
7. Fill paper lined muffin cups 3/4 full.
8. Combine the 2 tablespoons sugar and 1/4 teaspoon cinnamon and sprinkle over muffins.
9. Bake for 18 to 22 minutes.
10. Cool 5 minutes in pan before removing to a wire rack.

NUTRITION INFORMATION PER SERVING
Calories - 175
Protein - 3g.
Carbohydrate - 13g.
Total Fat - 7g.
Saturated Fat - 1g.
Trans Fat - 0g.
Cholesterol - 0mg.
Potassium - 54mg.
Sodium - 141mg.
Phosphorus - 85mg.

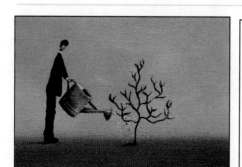

IMPORTANCE OF BREAKFAST
Chronic Kidney Disease and Diabetic patients should diligently eat their breakfast because a Harvard study found that people who regularly skipped breakfast had a 27% higher risk of having a heart attack than those who ate a morning meal. Still, as many as 18% of adults in the United States skip breakfast on a consistent basis. While sufferers of CKD and Diabetes often have very restricted diets, you can seldom go wrong with appropriate fruits in moderation such as blueberries, apples, cranberries, peaches, pears, grapes, blackberries or raspberries.

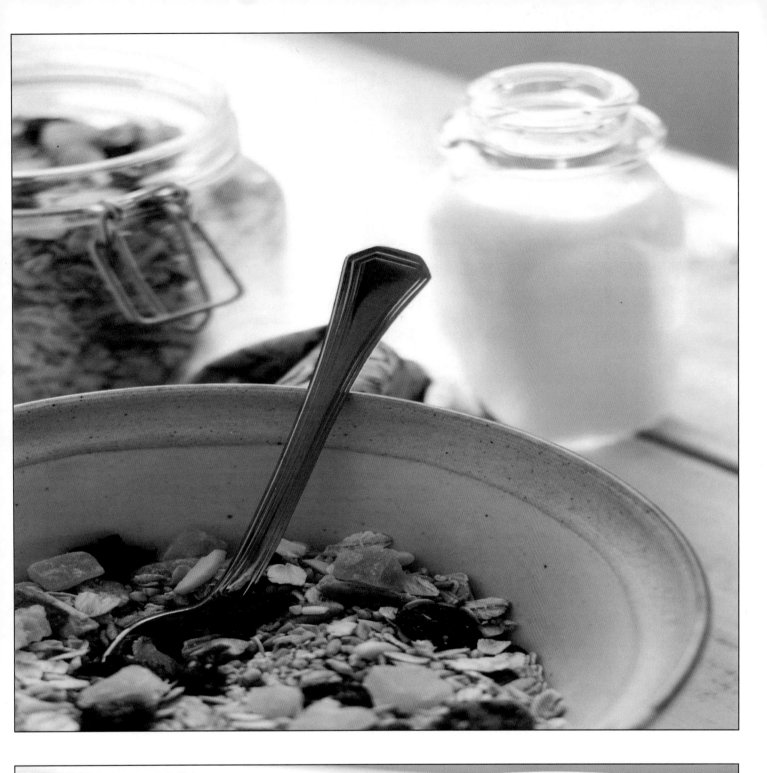

Milk Magic

Although many people with Chronic Kidney Disease and Diabetes are lactose intolerant, it is not an "all or none" phenomenon - most people are only a little lactose intolerant, and can still enjoy milk, yogurt and cheese. It is not necessary to completely avoid dairy products if you stay in close consultation with your healthcare team. In fact, dairy can play an important role for CKD and Diabetic patients because it is chock full of essential minerals and vitamins.

Cereals For Chronic Kidney Disease & Diabetic Patients

Next time you go shopping for cereal, look for the amount of Phosphorus and Potassium on the label. It is not always required, so if available the food manufacturer has added it voluntarily. In addition, look at the ingredient list and avoid products that have 'phos' food additives. High levels of Phosphorus and/or Potassium in Chronic Kidney Disease (CKD) patients can cause unhealthy nerve function, heart disease and Calcium to be pulled from bones and go into circulation. This can lead to Calcification of coronary arteries, cardiac valves, pulmonary and other soft tissues, and is associated with serious heart problems.

In contrast, Diabetics can eat all kinds of food, including many commercial cold cereals. According to the American Diabetes Association (ADA), diabetics should eat cereals with 3g or more of dietary fiber and 5g or less of total sugar. When choosing a healthy breakfast cereal, limit your intake of added sugar by skipping granolas and cereals with marshmallows, "frosting," dried fruits and chocolate flavoring. Also choose cereals that are higher in fiber because it is an important nutrient to help you prevent weight gain and heart disease, for which Diabetics and CKD patients are at increased risk.

Take a look at the Nutrition Facts on the label of "Ready-to Eat" cereals and select the brands lowest in Potassium and Phosphorus. Many cereals give the % Daily Value (DV) for phosphorus rather than milligrams. Try to go with those containing 10% DV or less. In general, cereals with added nuts or whole grain tend to have higher amounts of Phosphorus and Carbohydrates. You may also want to check the sodium concentration per serving of cereal because lower sodium choices will help with your blood pressure control.

Cereals that you may consider after talking with your Dietitian include Kix, Chex, Wheaties, Total and Cherrios.

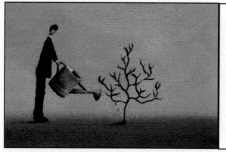

MILK ALTERNATIVES

While those with CKD and Diabetes may not be able to capture all of the health benefits from whole organic milk, they still can benefit from drinking effective milk alternatives. In recent years, the number of alternative milk choices in the market has grown significantly. Soy milk can be found in most grocery stores and is one of the most cost-effective choices, but products such as rice milk and almond milk have also gained in popularity. Bear in mind that all alternatives are lactose-free.

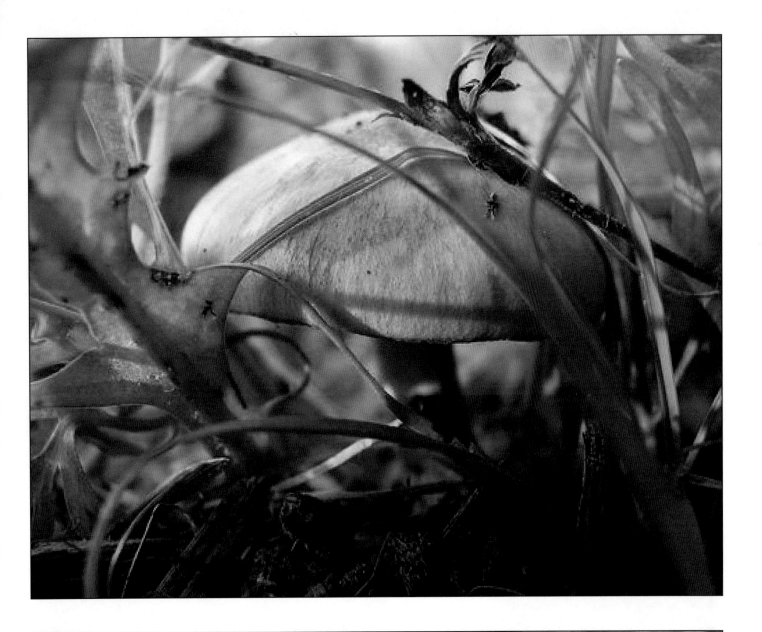

Forging A Healthful Diet

Looking to simply eat healthier? It can be tough to get the servings of vegetables you need every day. Yet, vegetables are full of vitamins, minerals and fiber, all of which are crucial for a healthy diet. We are even learning that the more vegetables you eat, the more diseases you ward off. When you eat the right kind of vegetables, you get a variety of health benefits and essentially no drawbacks. Here are some quick and easy ways you can "sneak" a few vegetables into your daily diet:

- When making an omelet or scrambled eggs for breakfast, top it with a bit of spinach.
- When preparing lunch, wrap your sandwich in lettuce instead of using two slices of bread.
- Use a blender or juicer to create a great blend of vegetable juice such as carrot, celery, beetroot, and ginger.
- Use the pulp from juicing vegetables and put them into pancakes, muffins or other baked goods for enhanced texture and flavor.
- Make a big pot of delicious vegetable soup that includes cabbage, bean sprouts, sweet pepper, broccoli, cauliflower, eggplant, onions, carrot, mushrooms, snow peas, and celery.

Delicious Greek-Style Marinated Mushrooms

INGREDIENTS	QUANTITY
Minced Garlic	3 Cloves
Extra Virgin Olive Oil	1/3 Cup
Red Wine Vinegar	1/4 Cup
Whole Coriander Seeds	1 Tablespoon
Dried Thyme	1/2 Teaspoon
Dried Oregano	1/2 Teaspoon
Freshly Ground Pepper	1/2 Teaspoon
Mushrooms	1 1/2 Pounds

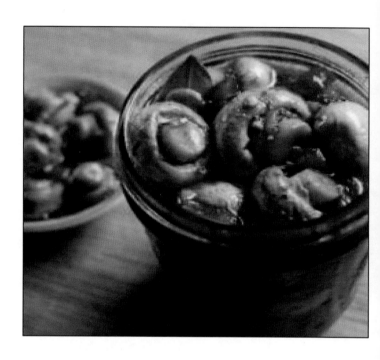

PREPARATION
1. In a large sauté pan, sauté the garlic in the oil for 2 minutes.
2. Add the remaining ingredients except the mushrooms; bring to a simmer.
3. Add the mushrooms; cover and simmer over low heat for 5 minutes, or until the mushrooms are tender, stirring occasionally.
4. Put the mixture in a glass bowl or jar. Cover and refrigerate 1 to 4 days.
5. Drain off and discard the

NUTRITION INFORMATION PER SERVING
Serves 10
Calories - 33
Protein - 1g.
Carbohydrate - 3g.
Total Fat - 2g.
Trans Fat - 0g.
Cholesterol - 0mg.
Potassium - 210mg.
Sodium - 3mg.
Phosphorus - 35mg.
Sugars - 1g.

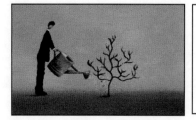

COOKING AT HOME

Studies have shown that eating at home is the single best way to promote a healthy lifestyle for those with Chronic Kidney Disease (CKD) and Diabetes. Beyond the advantages of a healthier lifestyle, eating at home can cut your grocery bill, improve the quality of your family time, and improve your selection of foods that you should and should not eat.

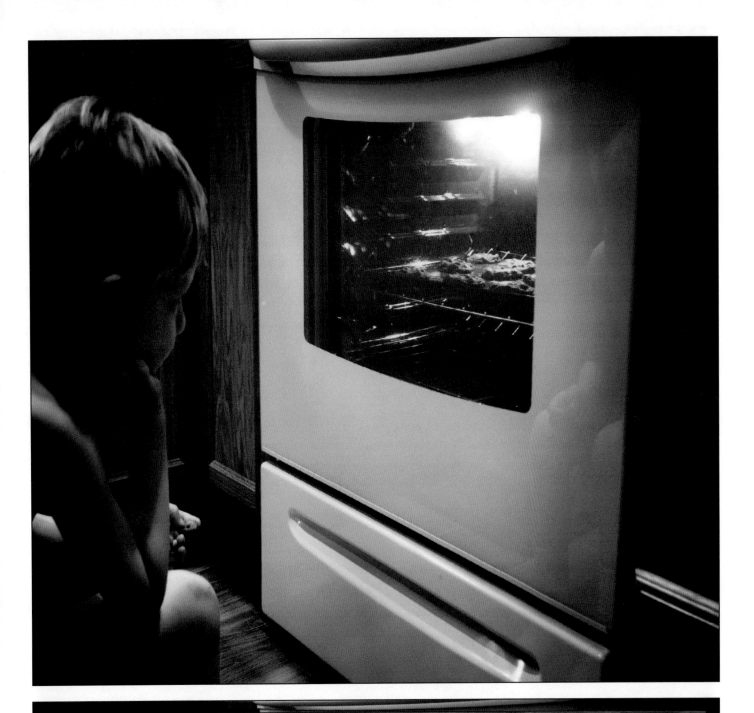

Diabetes Myth

The American Diabetes Association notes that, "Starchy foods can be part of a healthy meal plan, but portion size is key. Whole grain breads, cereals, pasta, rice and starchy vegetables like potatoes, yams, peas and corn can be included in your meals and snacks." Try to limit carbohydrates to about 45-60 grams per meal, or 3-4 servings of carbohydrate-containing foods. However, you may need more or less carbohydrate in meals depending on how you manage your diabetes.

Satisfying The Sweet Tooth

INGREDIENTS	QUANTITY
All-Purpose Flour or Almond Flour	2 1/4 Cup
Baking Soda	1 Teaspoon
Salt	1 Teaspoon
Butter	1 Cup
Sugar or Stevia (natural sweetener alternative)	1/3 Cup
Packed Brown Sugar or Ideal Brown No Calorie Sweetener	3/4 Cup
Vanilla Extract	1 Teaspoon
Eggs	2 Large
Nestle Toll House Semi-Sweet Chocolate Morsels or Cocoa Nibs	

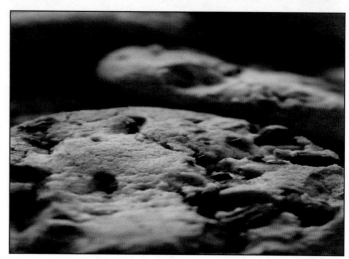

Image courtesy of Pink Sherbet Photography/photoree.com

PREPARATION

1. Preheat oven to 375F.
2. Combine flour, baking soda and salt in small bowl.
3. Beat butter, sugar blend, brown sugar and vanilla extract in large mixer bowl until creamy.
4. Add eggs one at a time, beating well after each addition.
5. Gradually beat in flour mixture. Stir in morsels.
6. Drop by rounded tablespoon onto ungreased baking sheets.
7. Bake 9 to 11 minutes or until golden brown.
8. Cool on baking sheets 2 minutes.
9. Remove to wire racks to cool completely.
For those with phosphorus restricted diets, consider grinding up phosphate binders and adding them to the outlined recipe. Also, by removing the egg yolk and using egg whites you will reduce the amount of phosphorus and potassium in the recipe.
Yields approx. 48 cookies.

NUTRITION INFORMATION PER SERVING
Serving Size - 1 cookie
Calories - 110
Protein - 2g.
Carbohydrate - 13g.
Total Fat - 7g.
Trans Fat - 0g.
Cholesterol - 15mg.
Potassium - 65mg.
Sodium - 85mg.
Phosphorus - 30mg.
Sugars - 4g.

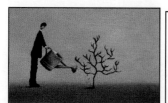

SATISFYING THE SWEET TOOTH
Like many foods on the kidney diet, some candies are okay in limited amounts and frequency. Guidance from your renal dietitian may help you learn which candies with a bit of chocolate or other limited ingredients you can eat periodically.

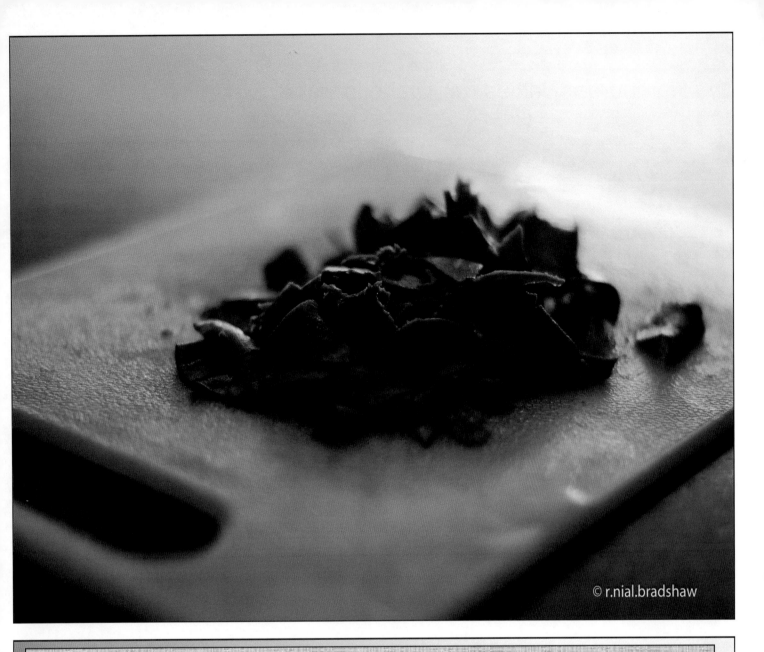

© r.nial.bradshaw

Dodging Foodborne Illness

Food becomes contaminated through a variety of mechanisms. Some of the things that can contribute to foodborne illness are: inadequate handwashing, cross-contamination, storage and cooking temperatures, and contamination of food by animal waste. Wash hands and surfaces often. Harmful bacteria can spread throughout the kitchen and get onto cutting boards, utensils, and counter tops. To prevent this:

- Wash hands with soap and hot water before and after handling food, and after using the bathroom, changing diapers; or handling pets.
- Use hot, soapy water and paper towels or a clean cloth to wipe up kitchen surfaces or spills. Wash cloths often in the hot cycle of your washing machine.
- Wash cutting boards, dishes, and counter tops with hot, soapy water after preparing each food item and before you go on to the next item.

Hamburger Patties For Diabetic/Renal Diets

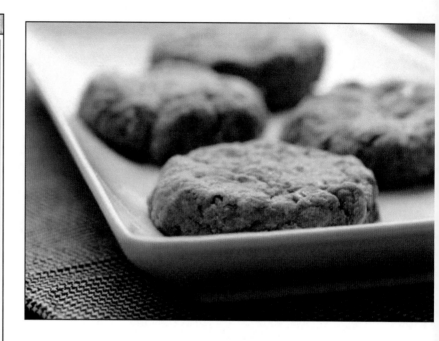

INGREDIENTS	QUANITITY
Lean Ground Beef	1 Pound
Low-cholesterol Egg Substitute	1/4 Cup
Nondairy Creamer	1/2 Cup
10 Low-Sodium Soda Crackers (Crushed)	1/2 Cup
Dry Mustard	1 Teaspoon
Chopped Fresh Garlic	1/2 Tablespoon
Black Pepper	1/4 Teaspoon
Dried Parsley	1/2 Tablespoon
Raw Onion	2 Tablespoons

PREPARATION
1. Preheat oven to 425° F.
2. Mix together all ingredients in a large bowl.
3. Shape into 6 hamburger patties.
4. Place patties in a baking dish.
5. Bake uncovered for 20 minutes.

NUTRITION INFORMATION PER SERVING
Serves 6
Calories - 188
Protein - 15g.
Carbohydrate - 7g.
Total Fat - 11g.
Trans Fat - 0g.
Cholesterol - 49mg.
Potassium - 231mg.
Sodium - 112mg.
Phosphorus - 136mg.

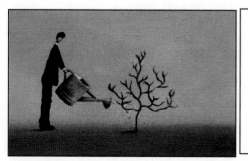

PLANNING AHEAD

If you are planning on eating and drinking more than normal, then make sure that you eat smaller meals and drink less earlier in the day. This will allow you to have a little extra at the party or during a special occasion and not feel poorly afterward. If possible, ask ahead of time which foods will be served at the party. That way, you can have a picture in mind of which foods you will plan on eating and which ones are not worth it. Make sure that you do not over eat or go too drastically off of your diet plan.

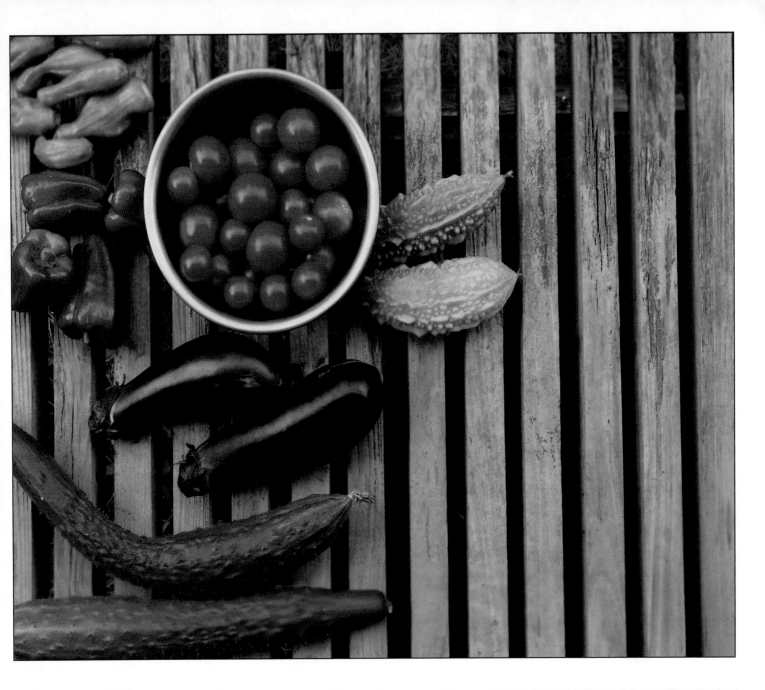

Food Blogging

To meet their restricted dietary needs, many Chronic Kidney Disease and Diabetic patients turn to published recipes such as on the internet, specifically Food Blogs. A study published in Journal of Nutrition Education and Development found that although food blog recipes are acceptable in calories, they are often excessive in sodium, sugar and fat. Given the growing popularity of online recipes, those with CKD and/or Diabetes should remain aware and alert to all recipes they utilize. KidnyBuzz.com offers daily recipes for those with CKD and Diabetes which meet patients' general Renal-Diabetic diet requirements (low sodium, low carbohydrates, low saturated fat, etc.).

Image courtesy of spinster cardigan/http://www.flickr.com/

Fun Quiz: The Taste Test

A. Bitter Food: You are craving relaxation

Bitter food makes your face jerk, twist and move so you are a magnet for movement and flow. This is important for helping people to "go with the flow" of life and relax. However, overeating foods that are bitter is very bad for people with CKD and may cause stress and tightness. Rather than indulging in excessive amounts of lemonade or sour candy find ways that you can sink into the moments of life and reflect. When you get a craving for bitterness try doing something to relax yourself, like deeply breathing, taking a walk, or meditating/resting. You may even want to try writing or painting to flow with your creativity!

B. Spicy Food: You are craving excitement.

Never quite settled, you feel the need for adventure and travel. Your mind has been active and restless and you are finding it difficult to be at ease. You live for new experiences and you are constantly seeking them. So you should try something new! Even if small, try to eat at a new restaurant or attempt to make a exotic dish.

C. Crunchy Food: You are craving more attention.

You are quite creative and experimental with a lot of great and useful ideas. Your confidence and outgoing nature allows you to offer many people great advice and you love the limelight. In fact you were probably born for it. Fulfill your need to be noticed by writing a blog post for the Kidney Community via KidneyBuzz.com or try volunteering and offering others help and advice.

D. Chewy Food: You are craving counterbalance.

You believe that a good life is filled with interesting experiences and nothing is going to rob you of them! A deep individual with a complex set of beliefs you may be feeling a bit unfulfilled, but you can see both sides of the coin in life and are good at staying balanced. Seek moderation and do not look for the extremes in life.

E. Sweet Food: You are craving comfort.

Above all else you value harmony and may be lacking comfort. You like to have as calm a life as possible and tend to be quite reserved, preferring to be around those who know you best. Although you are happy with the life that you have been given, you can use a bit more support from those around you at this time.

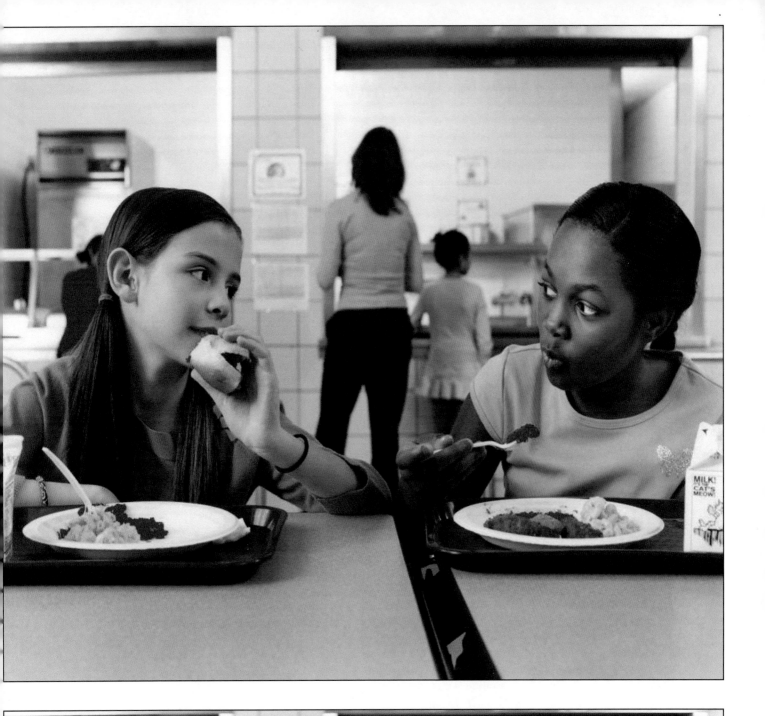

Controlling Diabetes

Controlling blood glucose levels and blood pressure are the most effective ways to manage diabetes. There is no generally prescribed diet plan for those with diabetes, rather, plans are tailored to fit an individual's needs, schedules, and eating habits. A diabetes diet plan must also be balanced. In general, the principles of a healthy diabetes diet are the same for everyone. Consumption of a variety of foods including whole grains, fruits, non-fat dairy products, beans, and lean meats or vegetarian substitutes, poultry and fish is recommended to achieve a healthy diet.

Tasty Chicken Pepper Bacon Wraps

INGREDIENTS	QUANTITY
Nonstick Cooking Spray	
Fresh Jalapenos Pepper	12
Fresh Banana Peppers	12
Boneless and Skinless Chicken Breast	2 Pounds
Sliced Onion	1 Medium
Bacon Cut Into Halves	12 Strips
Toothpicks	

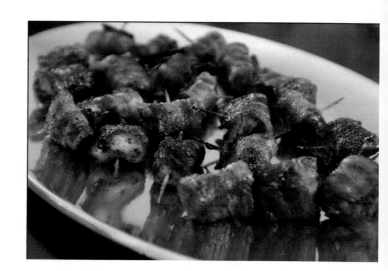

PREPARATION
1. Spray grill rack with nonstick cooking spray made for high heat.
2. Pre-heat outside grill on low or inside grill such as a George Foreman™ grill.
3. Prepare peppers by removing seeds from inside.
4. Cut long ways on one side of the pepper to split it open.
5. Cut chicken into 24 pieces, sized to fit inside peppers.
6. Stuff one chicken piece into each pepper.
7. It's okay if some chicken remains outside the pepper.
8. Place one slice of onion on top of chicken to cover.
9. Take bacon and wrap around pepper/chicken/onion and secure with toothpicks.
10. Use several toothpicks inserted in different directions to secure.
11. Place on grill.
12. Cook until bacon is crispy, approx 10 to 15 minutes.
13. Flip and rotate often to prevent flames from burning bacon as grease drips.

NUTRITION INFORMATION PER SERVING
Serves 24
Calories - 71
Protein - 10g.
Carbohydrate - 1g.
Total Fat - 3g.
Trans Fat - 0g.
Cholesterol - 26mg.
Potassium - 147mg.
Sodium - 96mg.
Phosphorus - 84mg.
Sugars -0g.

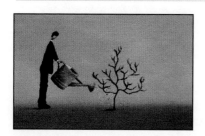

PORTION MODERATION
Milk products should be limited to two servings per day based on their phosphorus content and your diet restrictions. Dark colas should be completely avoided. Portion control should be adhered as well as being consistent with servings of carbohydrates consumed at each meal in order to maintain stable glucose levels.

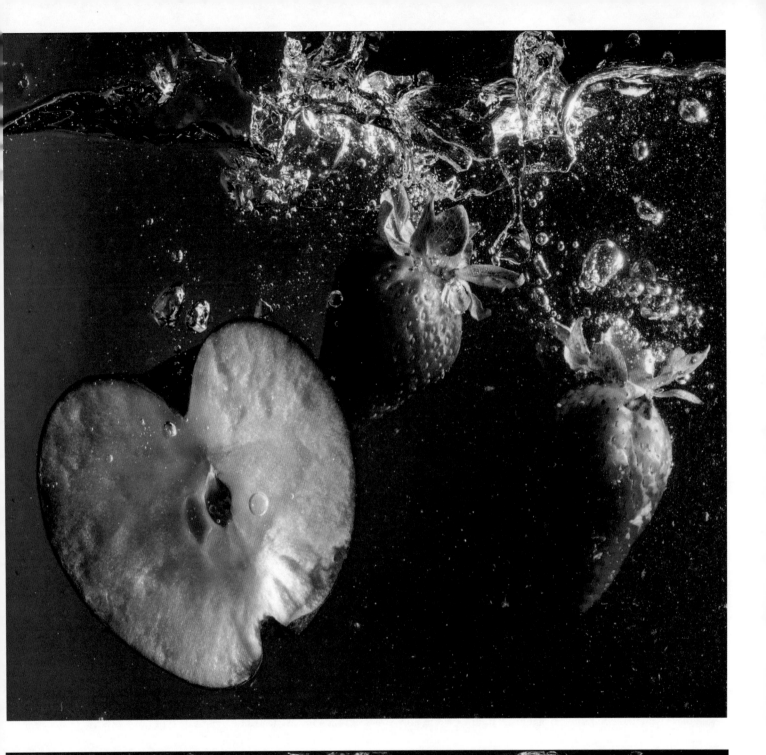

Staying Fresh

The chemical bisphenol A (BPA) is found in many kinds of plastic food packaging, such as some water bottles, food storage containers, sealing wrap and inside of food cans. The chemical has been associated with a host of health problems, including heart disease, diabetes, breast cancer, and infertility in adults, and attention deficit hyperactivity disorder (ADHD) in children.

Families who gave up canned foods and beverages packaged using plastic containers saw their levels of the hormone-disrupting chemical fall by 66%, a new study shows. All it took was three days a week of eating only freshly prepared, organic foods.

Grocery Shopping & Buying Right

Produce

Produce makes up an important and healthy portion of your diabetic diet. Produce items are low in calories and high in vitamins, minerals and fiber. Fruits contain carbohydrates and the American Diabetes Association suggests you limit your daily intake to three or four servings a day. Carbohydrates in food raise blood sugar. Fruits to add to your grocery list include small apples, oranges and bananas, pears grapes, berries, melon, pears and cherries. Vegetables also contain carbohydrates including peas, corn, potatoes and winter squash. Starchy vegetables can make a healthy contribution to your diet and should be added to your grocery list. Non-starchy vegetables contain only small amounts of carbohydrate and intake is not usually restricted. Try eating broccoli, green beans, carrots, leafy greens, green beans, mushroom, onions and eggplants.

Dairy Aisle

While some foods in the dairy aisle may be a source of fat and calories, by reading labels you can make the best choices for your needs. Healthy options from the dairy aisle to add to your grocery list include skim milk, low-fat cheeses, eggs, egg substitutes, margarine and nonfat sugar-free yogurt.

Meat, Poultry and Fish

Meat, poultry and fish do not contain carbohydrates, but can be a source of calories and fat. Choose more lean cuts of meat to limit your intake. Lean meat options to add to your grocery list include skinless white meat poultry, fish, beef eye of round, pork loin and lamb chops When looking at processed meats, like hot dogs and luncheon meats, choose items that have less than 3 g of fat per serving.

Canned Dry & Frozen Food

Grains and starches can be found in the canned and dry foods aisle. Starches and grains contain carbohydrates and intake needs to be controlled. Choosing high fiber starches and grains can help you better manage your blood sugar. The best foods to add to your grocery list include whole wheat pasta, brown rice, barley, dried or canned legumes, low-sodium canned starchy vegetables, whole-grain cereals and crackers, unsweetened canned fruits, low-sodium broth-based soups and low-sugar jellies.

Many items in the frozen food aisle often contain high amounts of sodium calories, carbohydrates and fat. You may consider adding frozen vegetables (without added sauces) and low-fat, low-calorie, low-sodium frozen meals. Try not to eat these types of foods very often.

Baked Goods

The American Diabetes Association says you do not need to avoid foods in the baked goods aisle, but it helps to make wise food choices and control the amount you eat. Whole-grain breads can be found in the baked good aisle and make a healthy addition to your grocery list. When it comes to sweets, go for small pre-portioned items like cookies, and try cake and brownies without frosting. Lower-calorie sweets you can add to your grocery list include vanilla wafers and angel food cake.

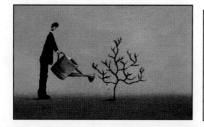

MANAGING YOUR THIRST

The best way to reduce fluid intake is to reduce thirst caused by the salt you eat. Avoid salty foods like chips and pretzels. Choose low-sodium products. You can keep your fluids down by drinking from smaller cups or glasses. Freeze juice in an ice cube tray and eat it like a popsicle, but just remember to count the popsicle in your fluid allowance!

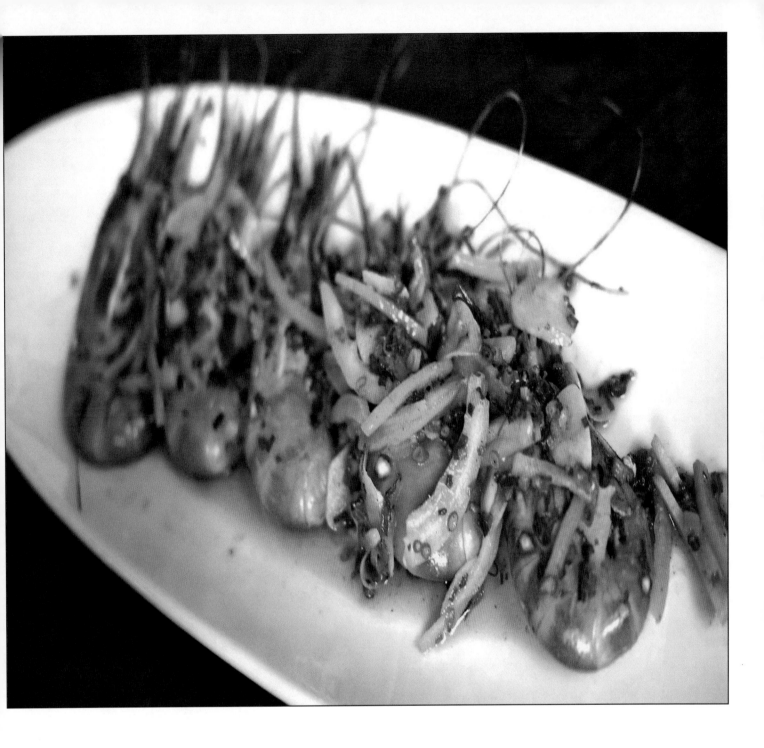

The Right Vitamin And Mineral Supplement

Vitamins and minerals may be missing from your diet because you have to avoid so many foods. Your doctor may prescribe a vitamin and mineral supplement. Do not take vitamin supplements that you can buy off the store shelf. They may contain vitamins or minerals that are harmful to your particular diet. You may be able to gain natural nutrients and minerals such as Omega 3, from sea food such as fish and shrimp.

Fish Cakes with Cilantro Pesto

INGREDIENTS	QUANTITY
Boneless and Skinless Wild Alaskan Salmon	6 Ounce Cans (2)
Lemon	1 Medium
Dry Breadcrumbs (Use Almond Meal as an optional alternative)	1/4 Cup
Mayonnaise	2 Tablespoons
Chopped Fresh Cilantro	1 Tablespoon
Ground Mace or Nutmeg	1/4 Tablespoon
Butter	1 Tablespoon
Pesto	To Taste
Olive Oil	1/4 Cup
Peeled Clove Garlic	1
Cilantro Leaves	

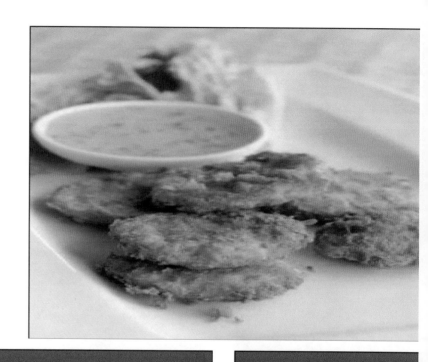

PREPARATION

1. To prepare salmon cakes: Flake salmon into a bowl, removing any small bones or skin. Cut lemon in half; juice one half and cut the other half into 4 wedges.
2. Add the lemon juice, breadcrumbs, mayonnaise, chopped cilantro and mace (or nutmeg) to the bowl.
3. Mix gently with your fingers until well combined.
4. Form into 4 patties 1 inch thick (use a scant 1/2 cup for each).
5. Let sit for about 5 minutes to let the breadcrumbs absorb the flavor.
6. To prepare pesto: Meanwhile, place oil, almonds and garlic in a blender and pulse to combine.
7. With the blender on medium speed, begin to add cilantro, a handful at a time.
8. Continue, scraping down the sides, until all the leaves are pureed and you have a thick paste.
9. Heat butter in a large nonstick skillet over medium heat until foaming.
10. Add the salmon cakes and cook, gently turning halfway through, until golden on both sides, 5 to 6 minutes total.
11. Adjust the heat and reshape the cakes as necessary.
12. Serve the salmon cakes with the pesto and a wedge of lemon.
Optional: Use sour cream (light) if cilantro pesto conflicts with your diet restrictions.

NUTRITION INFORMATION PER SERVING

Serves 4
Calories - 302
Protein - 18g.
Carbohydrates - 8g.
Total Fat - 0g.
Cholesterol - 33mg.
Potassium - 125mg.
Sodium - 180mg.
Phosphorus - 90mg.
Sugar - 0g.

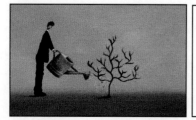

OMEGA 3 FATTY ACIDS

Eating fish 2-3 times a week helps treat inflammation because of the anti-inflammatory effect of omega-3 fatty acids in fish. Albacore tuna, herring, mackerel, rainbow trout and salmon are among the fish highest in omega 3s. If you do not like fish, consider taking fish oil supplements after talking to your Dietitian.

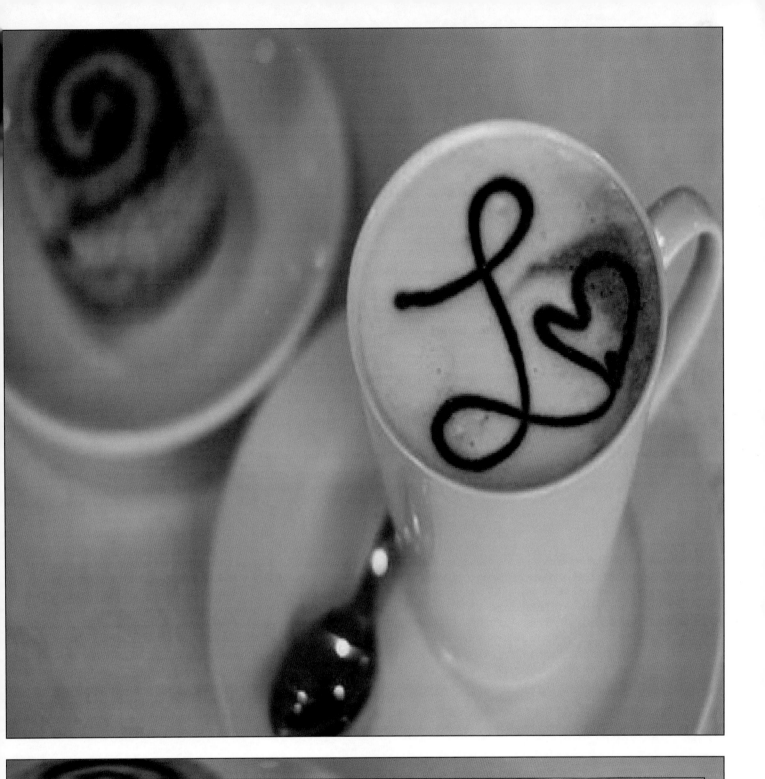

Drinking Coffee

Some say that coffee is good for Chronic Kidney Disease (CKD) patients while others say that it's bad. However, coffee in moderation is not bad for the CKD patients. If you are on dialysis then you should restrict your intake to 4 oz. to remain within your fluid restriction. Nephrologist, Dr. Shamik Shah, MD suggests, "As a general rule, I advise my patients to limit their intake of caffeine.

Warm and Delicious Caramel Protein Latte

INGREDIENTS	QUANTITY
Protein Powder	1 Scoop
Water	2 Ounces
Hot Coffee	6 Ounces
DaVinci Gourmet® Caramel Sugar Free Syrup	2 Tablespoons
Sweeten With Sugar-free Sweetener or Stevia.	To Taste

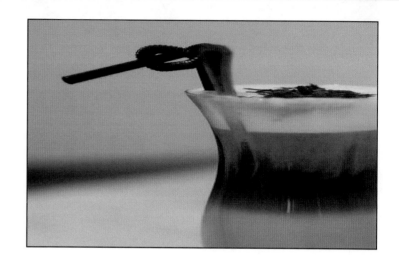

PREPARATION
1. Place 1 scoop of protein powder in a mug.
2. Add 2 ounces water and stir until protein powder is completely dissolved.
3. Add 6 ounces of hot coffee and stir.
4. Add 2 tablespoons of DaVinci Gourmet® Caramel
5. Sugar Free Syrup. Adjust to desired sweetness using sugar-free sweetener or Stevia.

NUTRITION INFORMATION PER SERVING
Serves 1
Calories - 72
Protein - 17g.
Carbohydrate - 1g.
Total Fat - 0g.
Trans Fat - 0g.
Cholesterol - 0mg.
Potassium - 214mg.
Sodium - 55mg.
Phosphorus - 75mg.
Sugars - 2g.

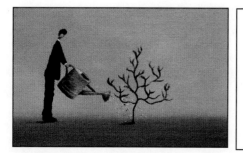

COFFEE AND YOUR HEALTH

Coffee contains antibiotics that may offer some cardiovascular protection, and research is showing that it reduces the likelihood of developing diabetes. The drink may also have anti-cancer properties as coffee drinkers were 50 percent less likely to get liver cancer than non-drinkers. Note that KidneyBuzz.com does not encourage beginning drinking coffee to gain new found health benefits. In any case, you should talk to your Dietitian before augmenting ANY part of your recommended diet.

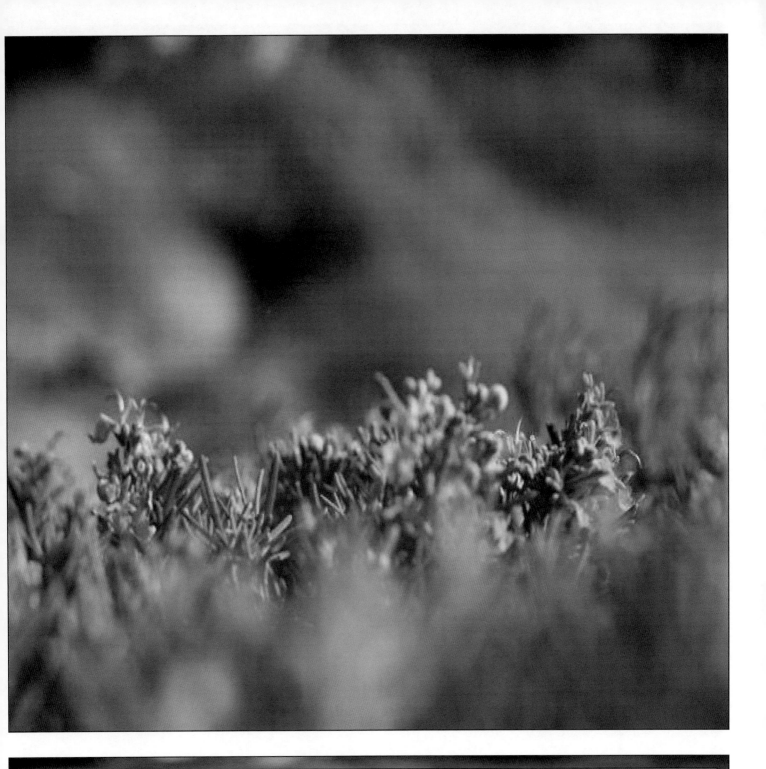

The Health Benefits Of Rosemary

The wonderful smell of rosemary is often associated with good food and great times. Now you can associate it with good health. There are substances found in Rosemary that are useful for stimulating the immune system, increasing circulation, and improving digestion. Rosemary also contains anti-inflammatory compounds that reduce the severity of asthma attacks and heart disease. In addition, rosemary has been shown to increase the blood flow to the head and brain, improving concentration. So, the next time you enhance the flavor of some special dish with rosemary you a making a health-wise as well as delicious decision.

Paleo Balsamic Rosemary Chicken

INGREDIENTS	QUANTITY
Organic Chicken	4 Pound Chicken
Balsamic Vinegar	1/4 Cup
Coconut Aminos	1/4 Cup
Fresh Rosemary	1/4 Cup
Organic Honey	1/4 Cup
Black Pepper	1/4 Teaspoon
Peeled Shallots	8 Shallots
Coconut Oil	1 Tablespoon
Minced Garlic Cloves	2 Cloves

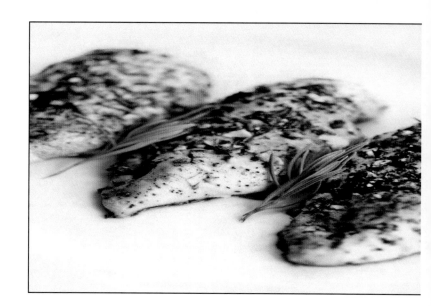

PREPARATION
1. Heat oven to 425 Degrees.
2. Combine balsamic vinegar, coconut aminos, rosemary, honey and 1/2 tsp pepper to a shallow baking dish.
3. Separate the chicken into pieces leaving the skin down.
4. Add the chicken and mix together placing the skin down.
5. Mix the shallots and oil and add to the dish on top of the chicken.
6. Roast the chicken for 30 min.
7. Flip the chicken pieces skin side up and baste.
8. Roast for another 20-25 min.

NUTRITION INFORMATION PER SERVING
Serves 5
Calories - 235
Protein - 7g.
Carbohydrates - 6g.
Total Fat - 15g.
Cholesterol - 119mg.
Potassium - 105mg.
Sodium - 8mg.
Phosphorus - 10mg.
Sugar - 0g.

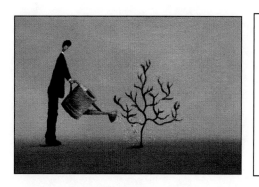

EATING CHICKEN IS RIGHT

The health benefits of eating chicken are enormous. It is a rich source of a variety of essential nutrients and vitamins which assist in strengthening the immune system of the body. Chicken is also reputed to be one of the safest meats available, as it is least associated with any side-effects of consumption. Many scientific studies have been conducted on chicken to assess its healthy properties, and most of the researchers have found very positive effects of the meat on human health including increasing bone strength, improving teeth health and cancer protection.

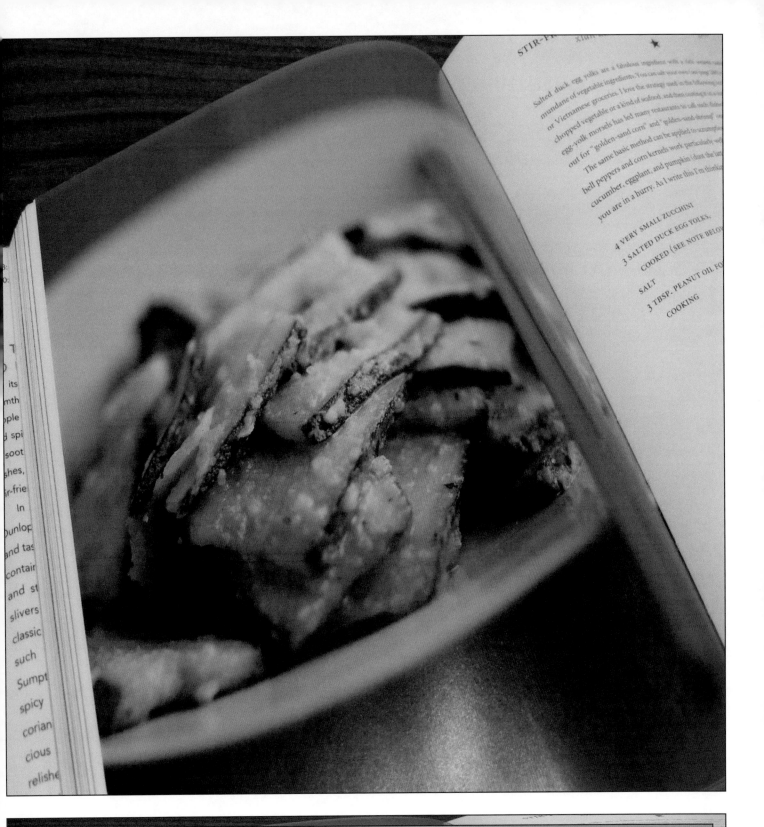

The "Miracle" Squash

Zucchini has been dubbed the "miracle squash" by well respected resources such as Health.com. It is one of the few squash that are low in potassium which is good for most of those with Chronic Kidney Disease. Zucchini is not only easy to grow, it also has lots of vitamin A, few calories, and is one of the most simple vegetables to cook. There are well over 26 ways to cook zucchini including in dishes that range from sweet to savory to spicy.

Image courtesy of FotoosVanRobin/ http://www.photoree.com/

Low-Carbohydrate Zucchini Pancakes

INGREDIENTS	QUANTITY
Zucchini	3 Cups
Onion	1/4 Cup
Almond Flour	1 Tablespoon
Mrs. Dash® Original Blend Herb Seasoning	1 Teaspoon
Liquid Low Cholesterol Egg Substitute	1/4 Cup
Canola Oil	1 Tablespoon
Salt	1/8 Teaspoon

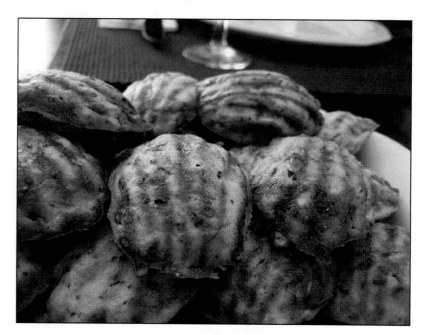

Image courtesy of infowidget / http://www.photoree.com/

PREPARATION
1. Grate onion and zucchini into a bowl and stir to combine.
2. Place the zucchini mixture on a clean kitchen towel. Twist and squeeze out as much liquid as possible.
3. Return to bowl.
4. Mix flour, salt, and Mrs. Dash® herb seasoning in a small bowl.
5. Add egg product and mix; stir into zucchini and onion mixture.
6. Form 4 patties.
7. Heat oil over high heat in a large nonstick frying pan.
8. Lower heat to medium and place zucchini patties into pan.
9. Sauté until brown, turning once.

NUTRITION INFORMATION PER SERVING
Serves 4
Calories - 55
Protein - 2g.
Carbohydrate - 4g.
Total Fat - 4g.
Trans Fat - 0g.
Cholesterol - 0mg.
Potassium - 198mg.
Sodium - 89mg.
Phosphorus - 27mg.
Sugars - 0g.

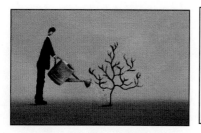

SQUASH IT!

With only 90-250 mg of potassium, summer squash (yellow squash and zucchini) is usually recommended for people with CKD who are on a low potassium diet. Though it is true that most winter squash varieties are high in potassium (250-445 mg), there are low potassium exceptions such as spaghetti squash with only 91 mg of potassium.

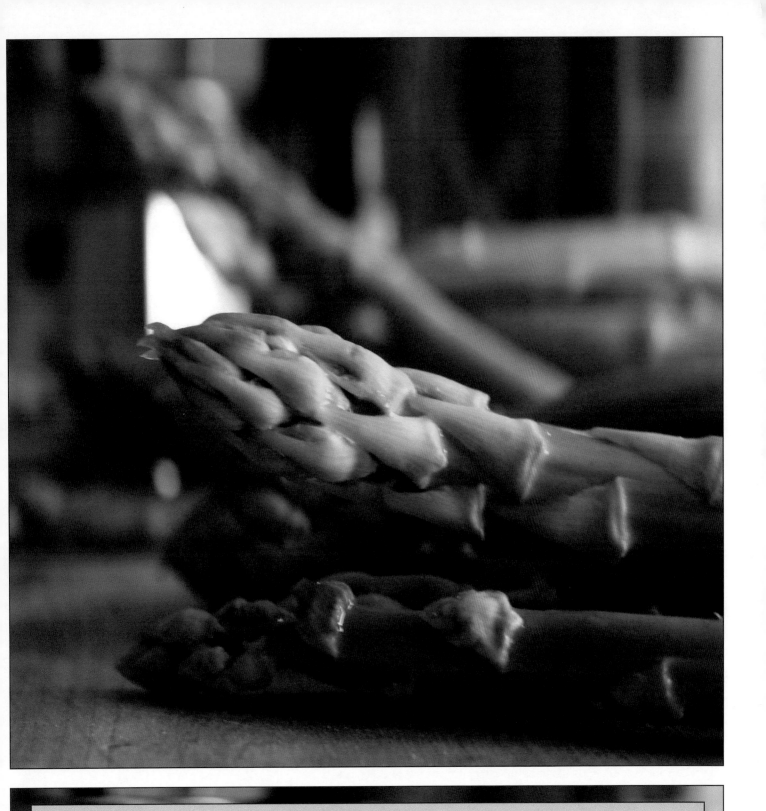

Asparagus And Insulin Production

The British Journal of Nutrition reported that eating asparagus can help control Type II diabetes. Researchers found that regular consumption of the vegetable can keep blood sugar levels in check as well as increase your bodies insulin production

Asparagus With Lemon Sauce

INGREDIENTS	QUANTITY
Asparagus	20 Medium Sticks
Fresh Lemon	1 Medium
Mayonnaise (Reduced-Fat Optional)	2 Tablespoons
Dried Parsley	1 Tablespoon
Ground Black Pepper	1/8 Teaspoons

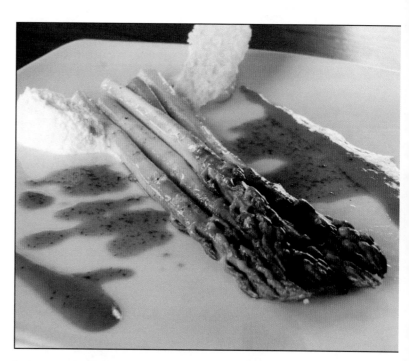

Image courtesy of Yarden Sachs/ http://www.photoree.com/

PREPARATION
1. Place 1 inch of water in a 4-quart pot with a lid.
2. Place a steamer basket inside the pot, and add asparagus.
3. Cover and bring to a boil over high heat.
4. Reduce heat to medium. Cook for 10 minutes, until asparagus is easily pierced with a sharp knife.
5. Do not overcook.
6. While the asparagus cooks, grate the lemon zest into a small bowl. Cut the lemon in half and squeeze the juice into the bowl.
7. Use the back of a spoon to press out extra juice and remove pits. Add mayonnaise, parsley, pepper, and salt.
8. Stir well. Set aside.
9. When the asparagus is tender, remove the pot from the heat.
10. Place asparagus spears in a serving bowl.
11. Drizzle the lemon sauce evenly over the asparagus (about 1-1/2 teaspoons per portion) and serve.

NUTRITION INFORMATION PER SERVING
Serves 4
Calories - 39
Protein - 2g.
Carbohydrate - 7g.
Total Fat - 1g.
Trans Fat - 0g.
Cholesterol - 0mg.
Potassium - 113mg.
Sodium - 107mg.
Phosphorus - 95mg.
Sugars - 0g.

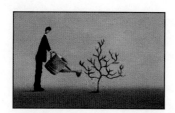

LEMON QUENCHING THIRST
Those with Chronic Kidney Disease must limit their fluid intake. You can use lemons to accomplish this goal. Suck on a lemon wedge. You can freeze it first if you would like. Also, you can add lemon to water and ice for a thirst-quenching effect.

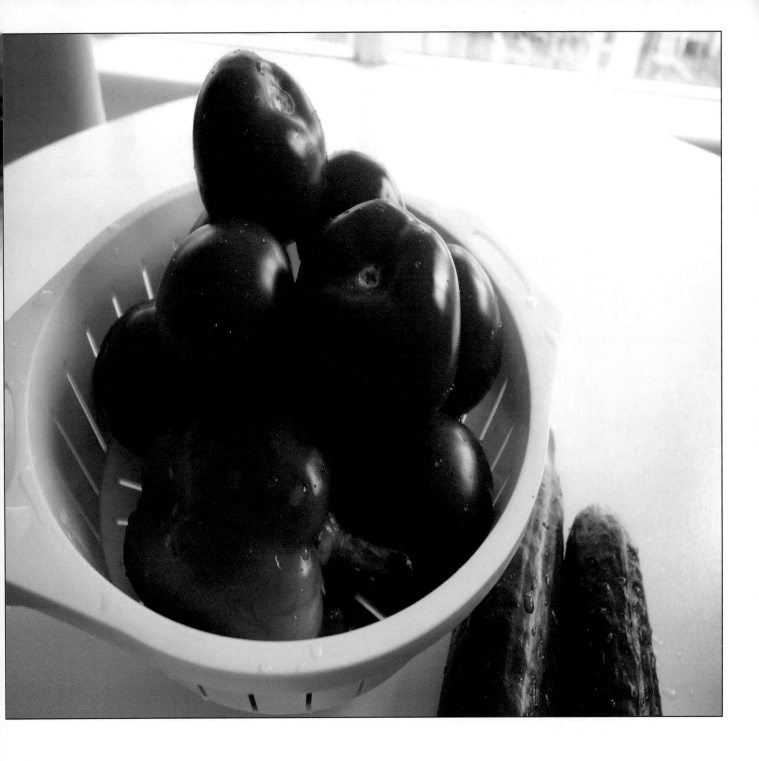

To Wash Or Not To Wash?

Many pre-cut, bagged, or packaged produce items like lettuce are pre-washed and ready-to-eat. The Food and Drug Administration (FDA) notes that if so, it will be stated on the packaging. If the package indicates that the contents are pre-washed and ready-to-eat, you can use the produce without further washing. If you do chose to wash a product marked "pre-washed" or "ready-to-eat," be sure to use safe handling practices to avoid any cross contamination.

Smothered Green Beans with Leached Potatoes

INGREDIENTS	QUANTITY
Trimmed Green Beans	1 Pound
Onions	1 0r 2 Medium
Leached Potatoes	12 Ounces
Freshly Ground Pepper	1 Teaspoon
Water	4 Cup

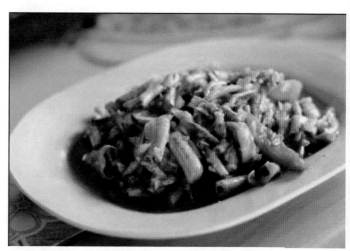

Image courtesy of rakratchada torsap / FreeDigitalPhotos.net

PREPARATION
1. Add beans, onions, potatoes, pepper, salt and water.
2. Stir well and bring to a simmer. Reduce heat to maintain a gentle simmer.
3. Cover and cook, stirring occasionally, until the beans are very tender, about 1 hour.
4. Uncover, increase the heat to medium-high and cook, stirring occasionally, until thickened and most of the water has evaporated, 20 to 25 minutes more.

If your diet allows, the dish can also include meat such as bacon. Simply, place a Dutch oven over medium heat, add bacon and cook until slightly browned but still soft.
Feel free to substitute other meats such as chicken if you cannot eat bacon.

NUTRITION INFORMATION PER SERVING
Serves 8
Calories - 88
Protein - 4g.
Carbohydrates - 7g.
Total Fat - 2g.
Cholesterol - 5mg.
Potassium - 160mg.
Sodium - 170mg.
Phosphorus - 40mg.
Sugar - 0g.

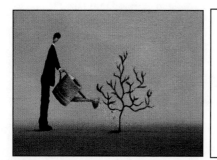

LEACHING VEGETABLES
The process of leaching will help pull potassium out of some high-potassium vegetables. It is important to remember that leaching will not pull all of the potassium out of the vegetable. You must still limit the amount of leached high-potassium vegetables you eat. Ask your Dietitian about the amount of leached vegetables that you can safely have in your diet. Specific steps include peeling the vegetable and placing it into water for a minimum of two hours. Use ten times the amount of water to the amount of vegetables.

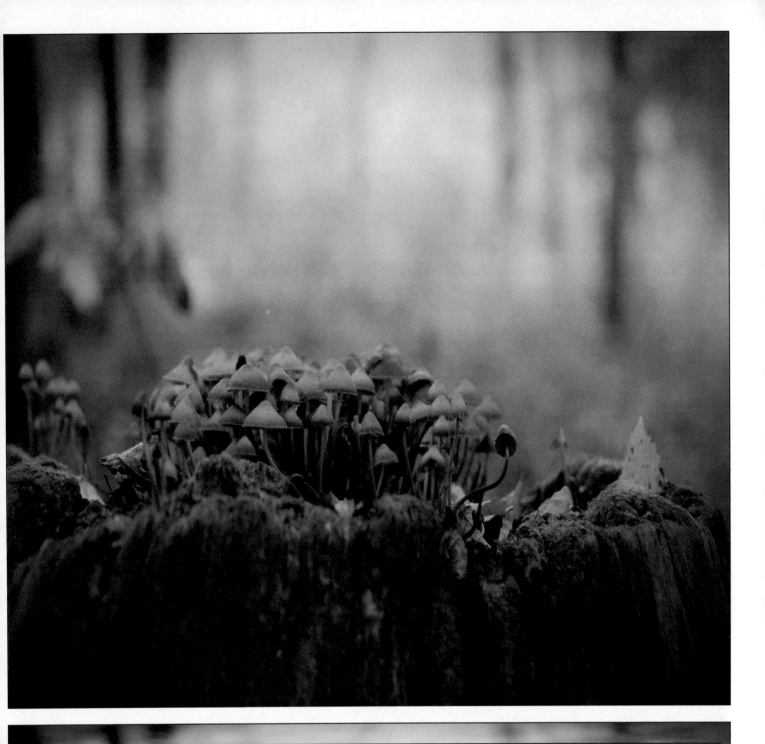

The Power Of Mushrooms

Many varieties of mushrooms contain "good-for-your-bladder" selenium and produce vitamin D when exposed to sunlight which is also good for those with Chronic Kidney Disease and Diabetes. Mushrooms are a good source of iron, plus, they are low in calories: Six medium white mushrooms, for example, have just 22 calories. Additionally, these veggies increase your immune system and metabolism.

Sautéed and Fluffy Mushroom Rice Pilaf

INGREDIENTS	QUANTITY
Low Salt Chicken Broth	1 Cup
Uncooked Instant Rice	1 Cup
Sliced Fresh Mushrooms	2 Cups
Thinly Sliced Green Onions	3 Onions
Margarine	1 Tablespoon

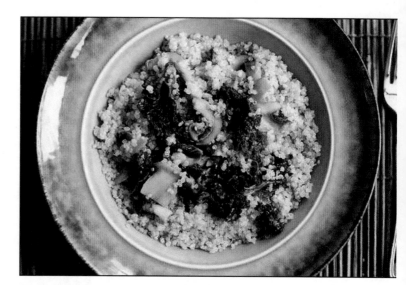

Image courtesy of SweetOnVeg/http://www.flickr.com/

PREPARATION DIRECTIONS
1. In a medium saucepan, bring broth to a boil.
2. Stir in rice.
3. Remove from heat, cover and let stand for 5 minutes.
4. Meanwhile, sauté mushrooms and onions in margarine and a dash of wine, for taste, until mushrooms are tender and liquid is absorbed (approximately 6 minutes).
5. Fluff rice with a fork and stir in the mushroom mixture.

NUTRITION INFORMATION PER SERVING
Calories - 72
Protein - 3g.
Carbohydrate - 13g.
Total Fat - 1g.
Saturated Fat - 0g.
Trans Fat - 0g.
Cholesterol - 0mg.
Potassium - 239mg.
Sodium - 145mg.
Phosphorus - 72mg.

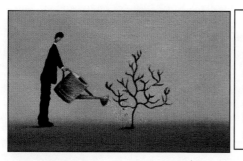

RICE AND BLOOD SUGAR

Eating for diabetics means selecting your foods wisely and choosing the best carbohydrates to suit your meal plan. Brown rice is an ideal replacement for high carbohydrate white rice. Every 1 cup of cooked rice is the equivalent of two carbohydrate choices on the diabetic meal plan. Each carbohydrate choice will cause a moderate rise in blood sugar, and brown rice is no exception. The added whole grains and dietary fiber will slow the process, however, causing a more gradual increase in blood sugar.

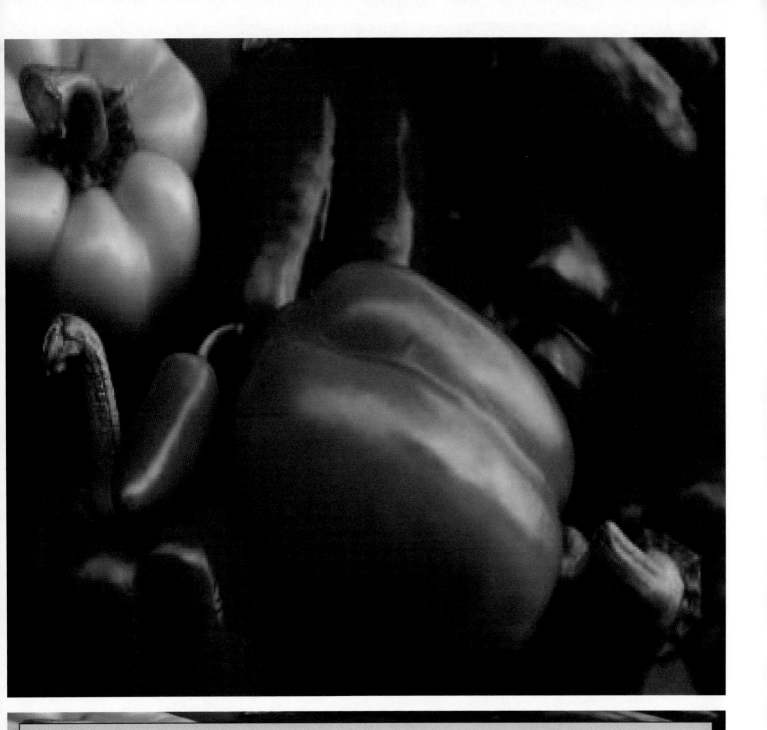

Naturally Found Vitamins

Many vegetables are good for Chronic Kidney Disease patients to eat as well as they can help improve kidney function in Diabetics. Davita.com recommends that they are low in potassium. Red bell peppers, for example, are a good source of the antioxidant vitamins C and A, B-6, folate, fiber and the antioxidant lycopene. Cabbage contains phytonutrients that help break up free radicals and prevent certain diseases. Cauliflower is high in vitamin C and fiber and contains compounds that can help improve kidney functioning. Onions are high in antioxidants. All these vegetables are low in potassium.

Healthy Raw Vegetables And Dip

INGREDIENTS	QUANITTY
Mrs. Dash® Onion Herb Seasoning	2 Teaspoons
Sour Cream	1/2 up
Celery	2 Stalks
Carrot	1 Carrot
Bell Pepper	1 Pepper
Cucumber	1/2 Cucumber

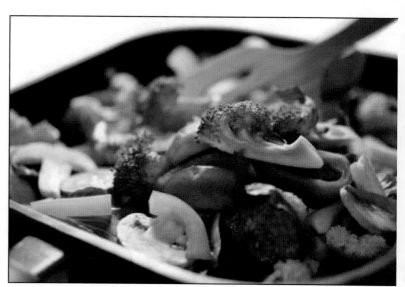

Image courtesy of amenic181 / FreeDigitalPhotos.net

PREPARATION
1. Combine Mrs. Dash® herb seasoning with sour cream and refrigerate at least one hour to blend flavors.
2. Cut each celery stalk in half lengthwise, then cut each into 4 pieces.
3. Cut carrot in half lengthwise, then cut into 4 pieces.
4. Cut bell pepper in half and remove seeds. Slice into 8 pieces.
5. Slice cucumber half into 8 slices.
6. Prepare radishes.
7. Place dip in dish and arrange with veggies on a serving platter.

NUTRITION INFORMATION PER SERVING
Serves 8
Calories - 37
Protein - 1g.
Carbohydrate - 3g.
Total Fat - 2g.
Trans Fat - 0g.
Cholesterol - 5mg.
Potassium - 140mg.
Sodium - 20mg.
Phosphorus - 25mg.
Sugars - 0g.

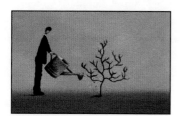

INCREASING DIET FIBER
To increase the fiber in your diet, eat more fresh fruits, raw vegetables, and whole grains. A higher-fiber diet may help lower your cholesterol, improve Kidney Transplant health and help balance your blood sugar.

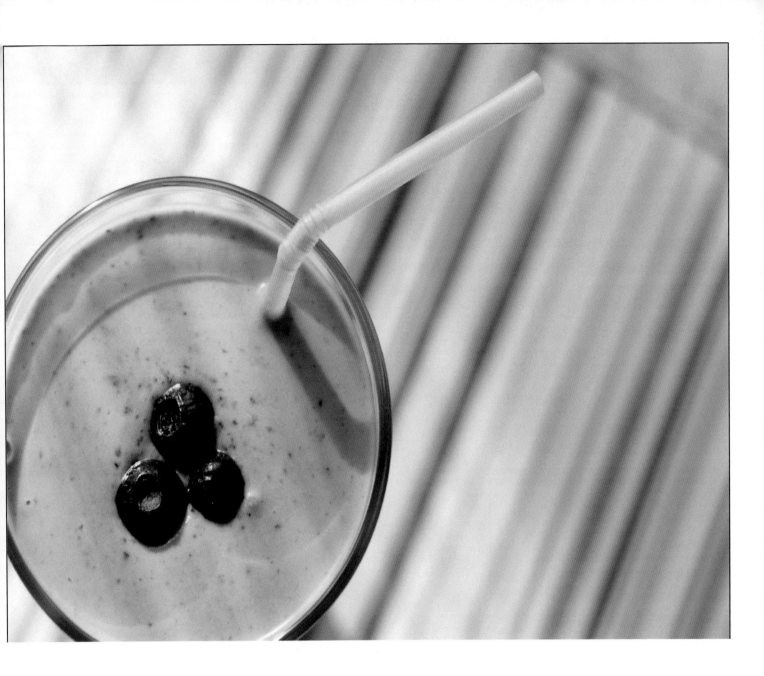

You Can Have A "Smooth" Life!

If you crave a sweet, cool and healthy treat, grab a smoothie. Smoothie shops like the familiar Jamba Juice and Robeks are ubiquitous these days, and for good reason. Smoothies are delicious, and many people even eat them in place of a traditional meal. But whether these blended beauties are any better than eating the same foods in solid form is open for discussion.

When looking at whether it is healthier to eat a smoothie or solid food, look at what you are eating. Many purchased smoothies are very high in sugar from sorbet, frozen yogurt or fruit juice. Thus, you should consider avoiding this extra sugar and choose an "all fruit" or "fruit and vegetable" smoothie made at home.

Image courtesy of Nomadic Lass/ http://www.flickr.com/

Simple Watermelon Renal-Diabetic Cooler

INGREDIENTS	QUANTITY
Crushed Ice	1 Cup
Lime Juice	2 Teaspoons
Sugar (Or Stevia)	1 Tablespoon
Watermelon Wedges	2 Small

PREPARATION
1. Place all ingredients except garnish wedges in a blender and blend for 30 seconds.
2. Pour into 2 small glasses and enjoy!

NUTRITION INFORMATION PER SERVING
Serves 2
Calories - 52
Protein - 0g.
Carbohydrate - 13g.
Total Fat - 0g.
Trans Fat - 0g.
Cholesterol - 0mg.
Potassium - 96mg.
Sodium - 1mg.
Phosphorus - 9mg.
Sugars - 2g.

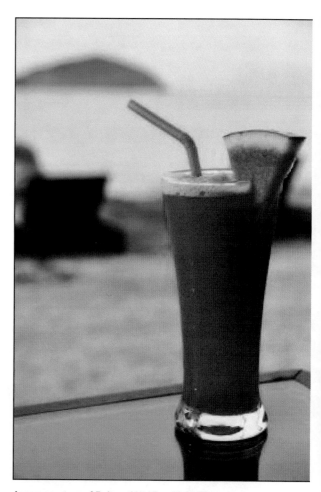

Image courtesy of Baitong333 / FreeDigitalPhotos.net

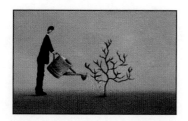

DRINKING SMOOTHIES
Smoothies are a great way to limit your empty calorie fluids, but don't forget to count them as part of your fluid and potassium allowances.

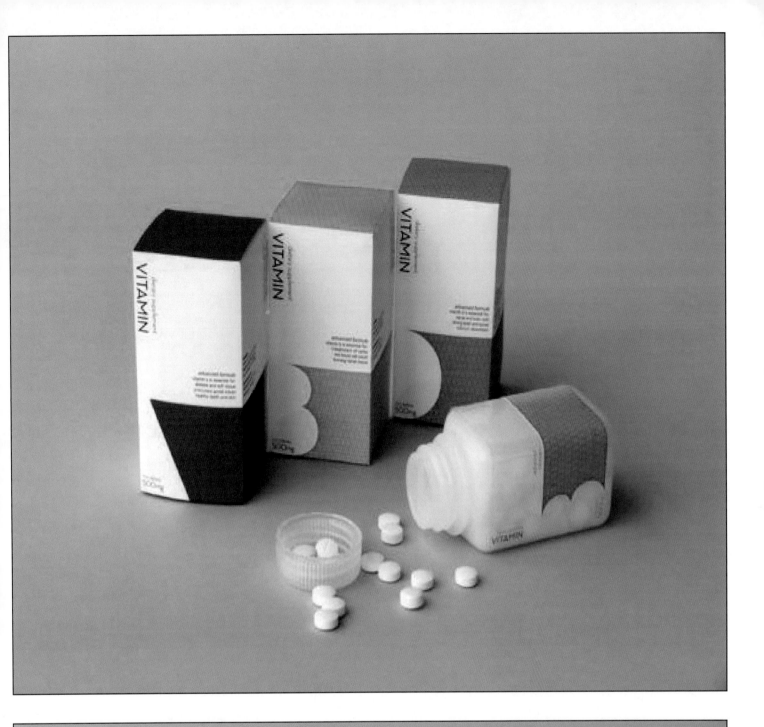

Taking Medication Properly

Medication adherence, or taking medications correctly, is generally defined as the extent to which patients take medication as prescribed by their doctors. This involves factors such as getting prescriptions filled, remembering to take medication on time, and understanding the directions. Poor adherence can interfere with your ability to treat Chronic Kidney Disease, Diabetes or other disease you may have, leading to greater complications from the illnesses and a lower quality of life.

Medicine Adherence Chart

Name:_____

Date:_____

Name of Medicine	Color	What Is It For?	Dose	How Often & What Time	Prescribing Doctor	Pharmacy Phone No.	Special Instructions	Refill Date
Aspirin	White	Blood Thinner	1 Pill	Every Day	Dr. Smith	555-555-5555	Take After Eating	9/12/14

Contact KidneyBuzz.com for a new Medicine Adherence Chart should you need a new one.

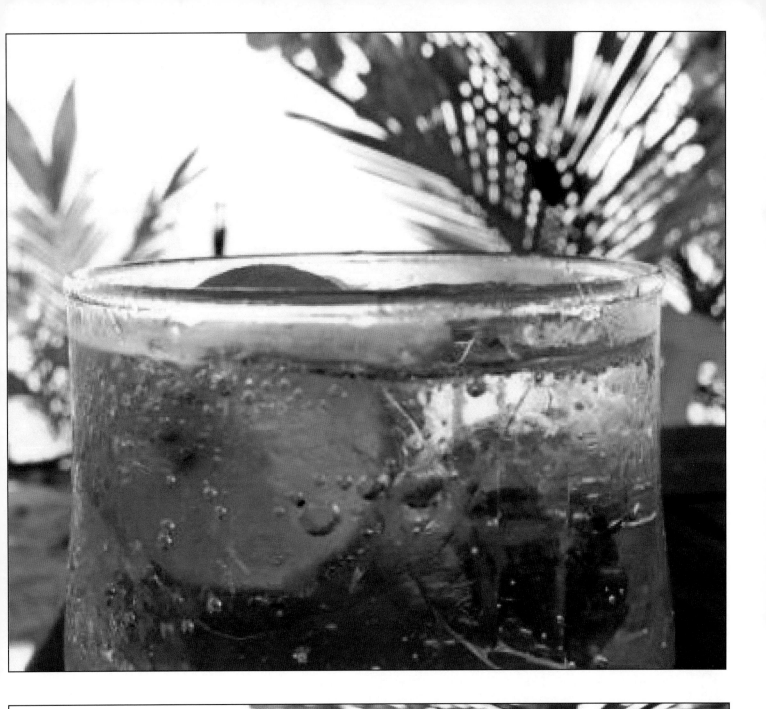

Drinks That You Should Avoid

The American Diabetes Association recommends that people with Diabetes and Chronic Kidney Disease should limit their intake of sugar-sweetened beverages to help prevent or manage diabetes. Sugar-sweetened beverages include beverages like: regular soda, fruit punch, fruit drinks, energy drinks, sports drinks, sweet tea, and other sugary drinks. These will raise blood glucose and can provide several hundred calories in just one serving!

Managing Your Numbers

Water Intake: You already know you need to watch how much and what you drink. What you may not know is that even though you are on hemodialysis, your kidneys may still be able to remove some fluid or your kidneys may not remove any fluid at all. That is why every person has a different daily allowance for fluid. Talk with your Dietitian about how much fluid you can have each day and fill out the chart below to

---

I can have _____ ounces of fluid each day.

Plan 1 day of fluid servings:

I can have _____ ounce(s) of _____ with breakfast.

I can have _____ ounce(s) of _____ in the morning.

I can have _____ ounce(s) of _____ with lunch.

I can have _____ ounce(s) of _____ in the afternoon.

I can have _____ ounce(s) of _____ with supper.

I can have _____ ounce(s) of _____ in the evening.

TOTAL _____ ounces (should equal the allowance written above)

Protein Intake: Before you were on dialysis, your doctor may have told you to follow a low-protein diet. Being on dialysis changes this. Most people on dialysis are encouraged to eat as much high-quality protein as they can. Protein helps you keep muscle and repair tissue. The better nourished you are, the healthier you will be. You will also have greater resistance to infection and recover from surgery more quickly.

Your body breaks protein down into a waste product called urea. If urea builds up in your blood, it's a sign you have become very sick. Eating mostly high-quality proteins is important because they produce less waste than others. High-quality proteins come from meat, fish, poultry, and eggs (especially egg whites).

High-Quality Protein Program

I will eat _____ servings of meat each day. A regular serving size is 3 ounces. This is about the size of the palm of your hand or a deck of cards.

Try to choose lean (low-fat) meats that are also low in phosphorus. If you are a vegetarian, ask about other ways to get your protein.

Low-fat milk is a good source of protein. But milk is high in phosphorus and potassium. And milk adds to your fluid intake. Talk with a dietitian to see if milk fits into your food plan.

I (will) (will not) drink milk. I will drink _____ cup(s) of milk a day.

The Renal/Diabetic Full Pantry List

Ask your dietitian how much potassium, phosphorus, sodium, liquid, and protein you should have each day. Your dietitian will tell you how many servings you can have from each of the food groups below. The approximate amount of these nutrients is listed next to each food group. Read the food label to find the exact amount.

STARCHE | These foods contain about 2 grams of protein, 90 calories, 80 mg of sodium, 35 mg of potassium, and 35 mg of phosphorus.

BREAD	RECOMMENDED QUANTITY
French	1 Slice
Italian	1 Slice
Raisin	1 Slice
Light Rye	1 Slice
Sourdough White	1 Slice
Small Dinner Roll	1 Roll
6" Tortilla	1 Tortilla
Hamburger Bun	1/2 of Bun
Hot Dog Bun	1/2 of Bun
English Muffin	1/2 of Muffin
Small Bagel	1/2 of Bagel

DRY BREAKFAST	RECOMMENDED QUANTITY
Cereal	3/4 Cup
Cream of Rice	1/2 Cup
Cream of Wheat	1/2 Cup
Farina	1/2 Cup
Cooked Grits	1/2 Cup

COOKED DINNER SIDES	RECOMMENDED QUANTITY
Noodles	1/2 Cup
Macaroni	1/2 Cup
Spaghetti	1/2 Cup
Rice	1/2 Cup

SNACKS	RECOMMENDED QUANTITY
2-Inch Unsalted Crackers	4 Crackers
Popped Popcorn	1 1/2 Cups
Unsalted Pretzel Sticks	10 Sticks
Tortilla Chips	9 Chips
Vanilla Wafers	10 Wafers
Shortbread Cookies	4 Cookies
No-Sugar Sugarcookies	4 Cookies

MEAT POULTRY & FISH These foods have about 7 grams of protein, 65 calories, 25 mg of sodium, 100 mg of potassium, and 65 mg of phosphorus. Do not use salt when preparing these foods.

COOKED MEAT	RECOMMENDED QUANTITY
Beef	1 Ounce
Pork	1 Ounce
Poultry	1 Ounce

FRESH OR FROZEN SEA FOOD	RECOMMENDED QUANTITY
Lobster	1 Ounce
Shrimp	1 Ounce
Clams	1 Ounce
Tuna	1 Ounce
Unsalted Canned Salmon	1 Ounce
Unsalted Sardines	1 Ounce
Crab	1 1/2 Ounces
Oysters	1 1/2 Ounces

EGGS	RECOMMENDED QUANTITY
Whole Egg	1 Large
Egg Whites	2 Large
Low-Cholesterol Egg Substitute	1/4 Cup

PRODUCE A serving of these foods contains about 1 gram of protein, 25 calories, 15 mg of sodium, and 20 mg of phosphorus. The amount of sodium listed is for vegetables that are canned or prepared with no added salt. Also, a serving of the below listed fruits contain about ½ gram of protein, 70 calories, and 15 mg of phosphorus.

LOW POTASSIUM VEGETABLES (Less Than 150 mg.)	RECOMMENDED QUANTITY
Green Beans	1/2 Cup
Bean Sprouts	1/2 Cup
Raw Cabbage	1/2 Cup
Cauliflower	1/2 Cup
Eggplant	1/2 Cup
Cucumber	1/2 Cup
Onions	1/2 Cup
Canned Corn	1/2 Cup
All Varieties of Lettuce	1 Cup
Small Raw Carrot	1 Small Stick
Raw Celery	1 Stalk
Fresh and Canned Mushrooms	1/2 Cup

MEDIUM POTASSIUM VEGETABLES (150-250 mg.)	RECOMMENDED QUANTITY
Asparagus	5 Spears
Broccoli	1/2 Cup
Celery	1/2 Cup
Mixed Vegetables	1/2 Cup
Green Peas	1/2 Cup
Snow Peas	1/2 Cup
Summer Squash	1/2 Cup
Zucchini	1/2 Cup

LOW POTASSIUM FRUIT (Less Than 150 mg.)	RECOMMENDED QUANTITY
Apple Juice	1/2 Cup
Applesauce	1/2 Cup
Apple	1 Small
Blueberries	1/2 Cup
Cranberries	1/2 Cup
Canned Pears	1/2 Cup
Canned Peaches	1/2 Cup
Pineapple	1/2 Cup
Strawberries	1/2 Cup
Tangerine	1 Tangerine
Watermelon	1/2 Cup

MEDIUM POTASSIUM FRUIT (150-250 mg.)	RECOMMENDED QUANTITY
Fresh Peaches	1/2 Cup
Fresh Pears	1/2 Cup
Cherries	1/2 Cup
Mango	1/2 Cup

DAIR The following foods have about 4 grams of protein, 120 calories, 80 mg of sodium, 185 mg of potassium, and 110 mg of phosphorus.

MILK	RECOMMENDED QUANTITY
Fat Free Milk	1/2 Cup
Low-Fat Milk	1/2 Cup
Whole Milk	1/2 Cup
Buttermilk	1/2 Cup
Chocolate Milk	1/2 Cup

DIARY PRODUCTS	RECOMMENDED QUANTITY
Plain Yogurt	1/2 Cup
Fruit-Flavored Yogurt	1/2 Cup
Ice Milk	1/2 Cup
Ice Cream	1/2 Cup
Cheese	1 Slice

FAT These foods have very little protein and about 45 calories, 55 milligrams of sodium, 10 milligrams of potassium, and 5 milligrams of phosphorus. Include healthy fats, such as unsaturated fats, which are listed below.

Oil	RECOMMENDED QUANTITY
Margarine	1 Teaspoon
Mayonnaise	1 Teaspoon
Sunflower	1 Teaspoon
Corn	1 Teaspoon
Soybean	1 Teaspoon
Olive	1 Teaspoon
Canola	1 Teaspoon

Printed in Great Britain
by Amazon